LIFE BEFORE DEATH

Reports of the Institute for Social Studies in Medical Care

The Institute for Social Studies in Medical Care was formed in 1970 as a development from the Institute of Community Studies, and its inauguration coincided with the publication by its Director Dr Ann Cartwright of *Parents and Family Planning Services*.

Further reports from the Institute for Social Studies in Medical Care will appear in this new series.

Medicine Takers, Prescribers and Hoarders
Karen Dunnell and Ann Cartwright

Life before Death
Ann Cartwright, Lisbeth Hockey and John L. Anderson

A catalogue of series of Social Science books published by Routledge & Kegan Paul will be found at the end of this volume.

LIFE BEFORE DEATH

ANN CARTWRIGHT
LISBETH HOCKEY
JOHN L. ANDERSON

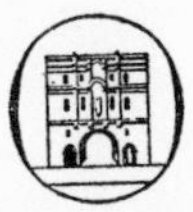

LONDON AND BOSTON
ROUTLEDGE & KEGAN PAUL

First published in 1973
by Routledge & Kegan Paul Ltd
Broadway House, 68–74 Carter Lane,
London EC4V 5EL and
9 Park Street,
Boston, Mass. 02108, U.S.A.
Printed in Great Britain by
Unwin Brothers Limited
The Gresham Press Old Woking Surrey

ISBN 0 7100 7540 5

Library of Congress Catalog Card Number 72-96768

CONTENTS

ACKNOWLEDGMENTS

A particular debt of gratitude is due to the relatives and friends of the dead who answered our many questions. They recalled many sad and poignant memories to help us.

Many others contributed to this study:

The district nurses, general practitioners and health visitors in our study and pilot areas told us about their work in caring for people with terminal illness, and the Medical Officers of Health and nursing superintendents in these areas facilitated our inquiries.

The Department of Health and Social Security financed the study and gave us additional information about the general practitioners in the study areas. Miss H. M. Simpson acted as liaison officer.

The Office of Population Censuses and Surveys—particularly Mr I. Hutchinson and Mrs Stobart—selected the sample of deaths.

The Queen's Institute of District Nursing seconded Lisbeth Hockey to work on the study.

The interviewers were Janet Baker, Millicent Bathgate, Stella Brown, Jill Cove, Beryl Davies, Kathleen Field, Connie Frost, Paula Garden, Ruth Harris, Ellen Latham, Anne Long, Mollie Richards, Angela Savage, Pat Tizzard, Muriel Toney, Mary Whitting and Kay Young.

Alison Anderson, Sarah Barnes, Gwen Cartwright, Linda Clayton, Peter Evans, Lisa King, Vic Lanser and Helen Ward did the coding. Joan Deane and Dorothy Hills punched the cards.

Wyn Tucker worked on the pilot studies and helped at the planning stages and with the recruitment and training of interviewers and the organisation of field work. John Bond also helped with the organisation of the field work and interviewing district nurses.

Jean Betteridge and David Sperlinger helped to check the report.

Peter Quince, Heather Robertson, Wendy Smith and Jane Thomas did the analyses. Ann Meade helped with the typing.

Queen Mary College, University of London, let us use their machines.

Members of the Institute's Advisory Committee, Abe Adelstein, Maurice Backett, John Cornish, John Fry, Austin Heady, Michael Heasman, John Horder, Margot Jefferys, Louis Moss, John Reid, Michael Warren, Peter Willmott, John Wing and more recently Albert Kushlick, helped at various stages.

Michael Alderson, Lance Burn, Vera Carstairs, May Clarke, Geoffrey Gorer, Tilda Goldberg, John Hinton, Bernard Isaacs, John Knowelden, Peter Marris, June Neill, Colin Murray Parkes, John Simons, Michael Wadsworth, Audrey Ward, Eric Wilkes, Brian Williams and Albertine Winner commented on the draft report and made many valuable suggestions. May Clarke also helped with the editing of Chapters 3, 9 and 10.

Ernest Gruenberg suggested the analyses on the proportion of hospital beds taken up by patients who will be dead within a year.

Howard Dickinson, Karen Dunnell, Chris Fitz-Gerald, Marjorie Waite and our colleagues at the Institute for Social Studies in Medical Care helped in various ways.

We are grateful to all these and others who helped, supported and advised us.

Among the three of us, the initial idea for the study was A.C.'s. L.H. did the pilot studies and preliminary work, collaborated on the design of the questionnaires,[1] organised and supervised the field work and commented on the draft report. J.L.A. helped with the analysis of the data, wrote most of Chapters 9 and 10 and part of Chapter 3, and checked and commented on the other chapters. A.C. wrote the other chapters.

[1] Copies of the questionnaires may be obtained from the Institute for Social Studies in Medical Care, 18 Victoria Park Square, London E.2. There will be a charge for photocopying when supplies run out.

1

INTRODUCTION

This study looks at the lives and care of a random sample of adults[1] who died. The common link between them was their death. But their circumstances, health and needs in the last year of their lives differed widely. This study gives a picture of the way our society cared for a group of people many of whom were old and many of whom were sick. The people were not included in the study because they were receiving help or because of their needs. They only came into the inquiry retrospectively and this way of identifying them determines both the strength and weaknesses of the study. Because they could be identified only after their deaths we could not collect information from them, the persons most concerned, whose knowledge of what happened was the most intimate and whose views on the adequacy, appropriateness and humanity of care the most important. Inevitably therefore our information is incomplete and may sometimes be inaccurate.

But because people were not identified by any recognition of their need for care, although many of them clearly had great needs, the study shows the ways in which a multiplicity of services function, or fail to function. It looks at the services from an unusual but highly relevant angle. Another advantage of this approach is the universality of the sample: we shall all become eligible for inclusion in similar samples at some time.

As we shall all die it is in our own interest to ensure that health and welfare services for the dying are humane and adequate. But possibly because we are embarrassed, inarticulate, or afraid about death we may tend to ignore these needs when we can, and consider them hastily and inadequately when they are thrust on our attention.[2] Death is less common than it was

[1] Aged 15 and over.

[2] For a discussion of this see Gorer, Geoffrey, *Death, Grief and Mourning in Contemporary Britain*, p. 172. Full bibliographical details are given in References on pp. 281–4.

a century ago: the crude death rate fell from 22·6 per 1,000 living in 1869 to 11·9 in 1969.[1] It is increasingly confined to the older members of the community: in 1869 over four-fifths of the deaths were of people under 65, in 1969 less than a third. This concentration of death among the elderly means that it is more often associated with infirmity and the need for prolonged care. Related to this there has been an increasing tendency for people to die in hospitals or institutions rather than their own homes. A century ago less than a tenth of the deaths were in hospitals, public lunatic asylums or workhouses: in 1969 over half the deaths occurred in hospitals. And even recently the proportion dying in their own homes has fallen quite dramatically: from 49% in 1954 to 35% in 1969. A number of changes have made it more difficult to care for people in the community. Greater mobility, smaller families and an increase in the proportion of women who work outside the home have made it less likely that people who are ill will be living with or near close relatives who are able to devote much time to their care. At the same time improved housing amenities and community services give some aid and support to people who are ill at home.

This study describes a number of aspects of people's lives and care in the twelve months before they died. It is concerned with their needs for medical, nursing and personal care, and the ways and extent to which these needs were met. It looks at the part played by hospitals, general practitioners, local authority health and welfare services, relatives, friends and neighbours. But who are the people we are considering? Before describing the methods of the study some basic information is given here about people who die, the causes of their deaths and the places where they die.

Who dies? What of? Where?[2]

Most of the people who die are old but men tend to die at an earlier age than women. These truisms are quantified in Table 1,

[1] See Annual Reports of the Registrar General for the different years.

[2] The figures in this section are based on data from Office of Population Censuses & Surveys, *The Registrar-General's Statistical Review of England and Wales for the Year 1969. Part I. Tables, Medical* and *The Registrar General's Decennial Supplement England and Wales 1961 Occupational Mortality Tables.*

which is based on the deaths of all people aged 15 and over in 1969 in England and Wales. Deaths of people under 15 accounted for 3·3% of all deaths that year, and three-quarters of these were of children under one.

TABLE 1 *Adult deaths by sex and age*

Age at death	*Males*	*Females*	*Both sexes*
	%	%	%
15–24	1·2	0·5	0·8
25–34	1·1	0·7	0·9
35–44	2·4	1·8	2·1
45–54	7·7	5·0	6·4
55–59	8·2	4·8	6·5
60–64	12·7	7·1	10·0
65–69	16·4	10·4	13·5
70–74	15·9	14·0	15·0
75–79	14·5	17·2	15·8
80–84	11·0	17·7	14·3
85+	8·9	20·8	14·7
Adult deaths in 1969 (=100%)	285,245	274,832	560,077

Whereas over half, 56%, of the women who died in 1969 were aged 75 or more, only about a third of the men who died, 34%, were as old. The proportions dying before the age of 65 were 33% for men, 20% for women.

In that year nearly two-thirds of the men who died were married at the time, compared with less than one-third of the women. Nearly a quarter of the men were widowed but over half, 53%, of the women. Ten per cent of the men and 15% of the women were single.

Although women were generally older than men when they died, and were less likely to have a spouse who might help to look after them, they were no more likely than men to die in a National Health Service hospital or institution for the care of the sick (see Table 2). However, rather more than twice as many women as men died in private hospitals or nursing homes and in other institutions. This suggests that their needs may less often be met by National Health Service hospitals or by informal care within the community. But less than 7% of all deaths occurred in other private hospitals or other institutions compared with over half in N.H.S. ones and over a third in people's own homes.

TABLE 2 *Place of death by sex*

	Male	*Female*	*Both sexes*
	%	%	%
N.H.S. hospital or other institution for care of sick[a]	53·9	53·3	53·7
Private hospital or institution for care of sick	1·7	3·7	2·7
Other institution	2·2	4·7	3·4
Own home	36·0	33·4	34·7
In other private houses or elsewhere	6·2	4·9	5·5
All deaths in 1969 (=100%)[b]	296,561	282,817	579,378

[a] Includes psychiatric hospitals and institutions.
[b] Includes deaths of people aged under 15.

Table 3 shows that people dying of ischaemic heart disease (mainly coronary thrombosis) were relatively likely to die at home. The proportion dying in N.H.S. hospitals or institutions was high, three-quarters, for the relatively uncommon causes of death: the 'other' causes which accounted for just over a tenth of the deaths. It was 80% of those with digestive diseases, 76% of those with diseases of the genito-urinary system but only 33% of the small group recorded as dying from symptoms or ill-defined conditions. These variations may be explained in part by different certifying habits of general practitioners and hospitals.

The small proportion dying in private hospitals or nursing homes was highest, one in twenty-five, for those dying of neoplasms (cancer) or cerebrovascular disease (stroke). A quarter of those dying as the result of accidents died in other places such as the street, an ambulance or at work. This proportion

TABLE 3 *Place of death by cause*

	Neoplasms	*Ischaemic heart disease*	*Cerebrovascular disease*	*Other circulatory disease*	*Respiratory*	*Accidents*	*Other*	*All causes*
	%	%	%	%	%	%	%	%
N.H.S. hospital or other institution for the care of the sick	58	38	58	47	59	52	75	54
Private hospital or institution for care of the sick	4	2	4	3	2	1	2	3
Other institution	1	3	5	6	4	—	3	3
Own home	34	47	30	39	32	21	18	35
In other private house or elsewhere	3	10	3	5	3	26	2	5
All deaths in 1969 (=100%)[a]	116,035	139,428	79,728	74,601	86,156	23,300	60,130	579,378

[a] Includes deaths of people aged under 15.

was also relatively high for those dying of ischaemic heart disease.

The main causes of death and the ways in which these varied with age and with sex are shown in Table 4. The information is well known but is given here as a background to the study.

Circulatory diseases accounted for over half the total deaths, the proportion rising from less than a quarter of deaths under 45 to three-fifths among those aged 75 or more. Ischaemic heart disease was the cause of more male than female deaths, whereas cerebrovascular disease accounted for more female deaths. Cancer was the second main cause, accounting for a fifth of all deaths, and the age and sex variations were in the opposite direction to those of circulatory diseases. More men than women die of cancer and the lowest proportion of cancer deaths was among people of 75 or more. One in seven deaths

TABLE 4 *Cause of death by age and sex in 1969*

	All deaths aged 15 & over	*Sex*		*Age*			
		Men (aged 15 & over)	*Women (aged 15 & over)*	*15–44*	*45–64*	*65–74*	*75 & over*
	%	%	%	%	%	%	%
Neoplasms (140–239)	20·6	21·8	19·3	25·0	32·0	23·4	12·6
Circulatory (390–458)	52·4	49·9	55·0	22·5	43·9	51·4	60·0
Ischaemic heart disease (410–414)	24·9	28·4	21·3	11·0	27·0	27·4	23·5
Cerebrovascular disease (430–438)	14·2	10·9	17·6	4·6	8·3	13·1	18·7
Other	13·3	10·6	16·1	6·9	8·6	10·9	17·8
Respiratory (460–519)	14·8	16·8	12·6	7·8	11·7	15·6	16·4
Chronic bronchitis (491)	5·3	8·0	2·6	1·0	5·5	7·3	4·4
Other	9·5	8·8	10·0	6·8	6·2	8·3	12·0
Accidents	3·8	4·0	3·5	28·9	4·3	2·0	2·4
Other	8·4	7·5	9·6	15·8	8·1	7·6	8·6
Adult deaths	560,077	285,245	274,832	21,701	127,898	159,144	251,334

was attributed to respiratory conditions. The proportion increased steeply with age, but chronic bronchitis was a much more common cause of death among men than women. Accidents, although the cause of less than one in twenty-five of all deaths, were the greatest single cause of deaths among people aged 15–44, accounting for over a quarter of these deaths.

Other data from official statistics show variations in mortality rates with social class, occupation and region. Table 5 summarises the class differences.

TABLE 5 *Social class and standardised mortality ratios*[a]

	Men aged 15–64	*Married women aged 15–64 (by husband's occupation)*	*Single women*
Social classes			
I Professional etc. occupations	76	77	83
II Intermediate occupations	81	83	88
III Skilled occupations	100	103	90
IV Partly skilled occupations	103	105	108
V Unskilled occupations	143	141	121
Unoccupied	63	45	115

[a] From the *Registrar General's Decennial Supplement England and Wales 1961 Occupational Mortality Tables*, p. 91.

The high risks encountered by men and women in Social Class V and the wide differences between those in Social Class I and Social Class V are striking. Regional analyses show higher mortality rates in the north and north-west and lower mortality in the south and east for all five social classes.

To sum up, official statistics show the age, sex and marital status of people who die, the causes of their deaths, where they die and their social class.[1] They do not tell us anything about the length of their illnesses and disabilities before they die, the pain, distress and symptoms involved, or the amount

[1] *Registrar General's Decennial Supplement England and Wales 1961 Occupational Mortality Table*, p. 516.

of care they need or receive. These are the concerns of this study.

Methods

The study was done in twelve areas in England and Wales. The areas were registration districts chosen with a probability proportional to population after stratification by region and type of area.[1] The interviewing was done during the six months July–December 1969, two areas being covered in each calendar month. In order to include deaths occurring at all times of the year, half the sample was selected from deaths which were registered three months previously and the other half from deaths registered nine months previously. Forty deaths were taken in each of the two periods in each of the twelve areas—a total of 960 in all.

Interviewers were selected and trained for this study with particular care. They needed not only the usual skills and techniques of interviewing but sympathy and understanding for bereaved people and the ability to express this without diverting or directing the course of the interview in a biased way. They also needed to be people able to cope with the emotional strains and demands of interviewing bereaved people. We think we were reasonably successful in finding such paragons. They tended to be rather older than interviewers on our other studies, fourteen of the seventeen being aged 35 or more, and a few of them had a nursing background. All were women.

The deaths were selected by the General Register Office.[2] They took a random sample of deaths of adults aged 15 and over registered during the relevant period whose usual place of residence was in the study areas.

The first problem for the interviewers was to find the most appropriate person to give us information about the last year of the person's life. Usually they first tried to contact the person who registered the death (or, more correctly, the person who informed the registrar of the death). If that person did not live in the study area, could not be contacted after several

[1] The way in which this was done and further details about the sample are described in Appendix I.

[2] Now the Office of Population Censuses and Surveys.

attempts, was too ill, old, or deaf, had since died or refused to help, they got in touch with the people living at the address of the person who died. The first questions were about the informant's relationship with the person who died and about any people who had lived with the dead person. On the basis of the replies the interviewer then decided whether the person they had contacted was the most appropriate person to interview. This was done on four common-sense criteria:

1. The amount of contact with the deceased—so people who had lived in the same household as the person who died usually took precedence over people living elsewhere.
2. The relationship with the person who died—here, other things being equal, the order of priority was spouse, son or daughter, parent, brother or sister, son-in-law or daughter-in-law, brother-in-law or sister-in-law, other relatives, friends, neighbours or others.
3. The amount of care the person gave—so female relatives were usually preferred to male relatives of the same 'degree'.
4. Availability, willingness and suitability for interview.

If the person initially approached turned out to be the appropriate person the interviewer carried on with the interview. If it was someone living in another household they found out the new address but asked the person they had contacted initially a few basic questions in case the other person proved unwilling or unable to help. If the appropriate person was someone else in the same household as the first person approached then the interviewer made arrangements to see the other person either then or at another time but did not ask the initial contact for any more information.

Questionnaires were completed for 785, 82%, of the deaths. Some incomplete data were obtained for another thirty-two, 3%. No suitable person able and willing to help was found for the remaining 15%. Reasons for the failures are shown in Table 6.

The most common reason for failure was refusal. Because of this the sample may be biased away from deaths that were particularly upsetting to the bereaved relatives. For example, one woman who had registered her mother's death said: 'I don't think I can face the details. I weep at the thought of it.

Mother was all I had. I had a terrible time looking after her.' When asked if there was anyone else who could help us she replied: 'There's no other relative. I had no one. I had to manage alone.' The other main reason for failure was that there was no one living in the area who could help. Among the

TABLE 6 *Reasons for failure*

	Complete failures	*Partial failures*	*All failures*
No one living in the area who could help	43	10	53
Refusal	81	15	96
Person temporarily away	7	4	11
Address of relevant person unknown or refused	3	3	6
Other reason	9	—	9
Total	143	32	175

complete failures there were twenty-three instances when a suitable person had existed but had since moved out of the area or died. In another 18 there appeared to be no relevant person who had had sufficient contact with the dead person to help us. For instance the death of a woman of 48 in a road accident had been registered by the coroner. Her house in Birmingham was now empty. Neighbours said she had lived alone but they did not know her personally. One neighbour remembered reading in the paper that her relatives lived in Nottingham. Another woman of 79 had died in hospital of congestive heart failure in the Isle of Wight. A son in Exeter had registered her death. A neighbour who knew her only slightly said there was no one on the island related to her.

The extent to which these failures bias our results is discussed in detail in Appendix I. The main conclusions are that interviews were more often completed for working- than for middle-class people,[1] 85% compared with 78%. The response was slightly better in the north, 84%, than in the south, 79%.[2]

There did not appear to be any significant bias[3] in relation to the dead person's age, sex, or cause of death. Neither was there any difference in the response rate when we tried to interview relatives three months or nine months after the death.

But there was some suggestion that, not unexpectedly, we were less likely to get a complete interview when the person who died had no close relative. The response rate was higher when the person died in his own or someone else's home than when he died in a hospital, other institution or elsewhere: 85% against 80%. It was also higher when the death was registered by a husband, wife, son or daughter than by some other person or relative: 84% compared with 78%.

How representative is our sample of deaths? Comparison of the initial sample of deaths with all adult deaths in England and Wales during 1969 shows that the sample contained a relatively low proportion of people aged 75 or more and a high proportion of deaths attributed to cancer. In addition the sample included a low proportion of hospital deaths and a correspondingly high proportion of home deaths: 40% of the sample deaths took place in people's own homes compared with 35% of all deaths in 1969. The details and possible reasons for these biases are discussed in Appendix I which also shows their effect. The main implications are that the sample contained an excess of married people and a deficit of widowed or separated people. The impact of these differences on reported symptoms, help and care appears to be small. The report is therefore based on the straight sample and no attempt has been made (except in Appendix I) to correct for these biases.

When the most appropriate person to interview had been located the main interview started with questions about the health of the person who died in the twelve months before death. Respondents were asked about the medical care given by hospitals and by general practitioners. Information was

[1] This was based on the occupation recorded on the death certificate. The 'middle class' have been taken as those in the Registrar General's social classes I, II and III non-manual and the 'working class' as III manual, IV and V. General Register Office, *Classification of Occupations 1966*.

[2] The north/south division was taken at the Bristol/Wash line.

[3] For a discussion of statistical significance, see Appendix VIII.

obtained about the dead person's household arrangements in the last year and any changes in these because of ill health or old age. We then asked about the symptoms he had, the help and equipment he needed and the expenditure incurred in caring for him at home. After that there was a series of questions about the relatives, friends and other people who helped.

The last section dealt with the impact on the respondent, as well as the person who died, of that final year. It focused on the information both had about the condition the person died of, the probable outcome, and the contribution of various people to their knowledge. It also covered details of the death, whether it was felt to have occurred in the most appropriate place—home or hospital—who was present, and the effect of the death on the respondent.

Many of the questions asked for much detail, so the interviews were often quite long. However, 18% lasted less than an hour: nearly half of these related to people under 65 who had died unexpectedly or to people who had been in a hospital or institution for the last year of their lives and so did not need any care at home during that time. Most of the interviews, 60%, lasted between one and two hours, 22% longer. In 68% of the interviews the respondent was the only person present; but other relatives were present in 29%, friends or neighbours in 3%.

Table 7 shows the respondent's relationship to the deceased. Husbands, wives, sons or daughters were the informants in just over two-thirds of all the interviews, other relatives in a fifth and friends, neighbours or officials in a tenth. Close relatives were less likely to be interviewed about older people and about people living on their own or with unrelated people. This is discussed in Appendix V and some attempt is made to assess the effect of interviewing close or more distant relatives. The data support the theory that close relatives may be more aware of people's needs and distress and that when we were able to interview only people less closely connected with the person who died their problems may have been underestimated.

As well as interviewing relatives we wanted to find out about the views and problems faced by general practitioners looking after terminally ill patients. Eighty-one of the 817[1] people who

[1] The 785 for whom a full interview was obtained and the thirty-two for whom a shorter interview was completed.

died had been in a hospital or an institution for a year or more. We asked the people we saw about the general practitioner of the other 736.[1] Two respondents refused to tell us the name and twenty-nine gave us inadequate or incorrect information so that we were unable to trace the doctors. Sixteen gave us

TABLE 7 *Respondent's relationship to deceased*

Relationship of respondent	*Sex of deceased* Male	*Sex of deceased* Female	*Completed sample*
	%	%	%
Husband/wife	49	26	39
Son	7	7	7
Daughter	17	30	23
Brother (-in-law)/sister (-in-law)	6	11	8
Son-in-law/daughter-in-law	6	7	7
Other relatives	6	7	6
Friend/neighbour	6	8	7
Official	3	4	3
Number of deaths (=100%)	418	367	785

names of doctors who had died, retired or moved from the areas. The remaining 689 gave us the names of 411 doctors and of these, 323, 79%, filled in a postal questionnaire or were interviewed.[2]

Doctors were asked about the difficulties of obtaining hospital admission for various sorts of people with terminal conditions, their relationship with hospital staff and district nurses, their views on the adequacy of local authority services, their attitudes to telling patients that they were dying, and about problems of caring for the terminally ill in the community rather than in hospital. They were not asked about individual patients in the sample.[3]

[1] Question 19: 'Could you tell me the name and address of ——'s general practitioner?'

[2] We tried to interview a random one in five of the doctors and sent postal questionnaires to the other four-fifths. Details of the sample of general practitioners are in Appendix II.

[3] At the pilot stage of the inquiry we attempted to ask general practitioners about specific problems related to individual patients. But the patients' records

Others who can play an important part in the care of people in their homes are district nurses and health visitors. All the Medical Officers of Health covering the twelve study areas agreed that we could ask the district nurses and health visitors working in the study districts about their views and the care and help they gave to the dying and to the bereaved. Five hundred and thirty-two district nurses were identified and 508, 95%, interviewed. Seventy-six health visitors in the study areas were involved in the care of terminally ill or bereaved people and seventy-five of them were seen. In addition to answering general questions about the problems involved in caring for terminally ill patients in their own homes, nurses and health visitors were asked about any care they had given to the individual people in our sample of deaths. One hundred and ninety-five patients were identified as having been given care by one or more of the district nurses or health visitors we interviewed and questionnaires were completed about all of them.

The book

The central part of the book, Chapters 4–8, is about the different types of care from hospitals, general practitioners, district nurses, other community services and that given by relatives, friends and neighbours. It describes the sort of help given and the attitudes and views of some of the people giving help—doctors, nurses and relatives.

Later chapters discuss the awareness of dying of both the patient and his relatives, the actual death and bereavement, and social class and area variations in needs and care.

Before looking in detail at the different sources of help, the next two chapters attempt to put them into perspective: Chapter 2 by giving background information about people's needs and care in the year before they died, and Chapter 3 by describing the experiences of particular types of people.

had generally been returned to the Executive Council and it was found that the information doctors were able to give us without these notes was unreliable.

2

NEEDS AND CARE IN THE LAST YEAR OF LIFE

What restrictions, pain and distress do people have to contend with during the last year of their lives? What kinds of help do they need? Who helps them? Where do people live during this time? Who lives with them? This chapter starts by describing the circumstances of death and then goes on to try and answer these questions.

Circumstances of death

How many people die suddenly without any previous illness or restrictions? We asked respondents whether, as far as they were concerned the person's death was expected. If the answer was 'no', we asked if it was completely unexpected with no previous illness or warning at all. Over half, 56%, of the respondents said the death was expected, one in ten that it was not and a third were uncertain or said there had been some illness or warning so that it was neither entirely unexpected nor expected.

> 'Not really expected. She'd spoken of this before—in fact she said a few days before what would we do if she did. I said we needed her. I didn't expect her to do it. She had two nervous breakdowns, one ten years ago and one two years ago. She took an overdose of pills. She'd been taking drugs for fifteen years for nerves so you don't expect this to happen.'

> 'Not then—though he'd been very ill for years. He'd been up and down for seven years and then one morning he asked me for a drink and died—heart failure.'

To some extent we were asking people an unrealistic question.

Everyone is expected to die sooner or later. The length of time over which a death was expected clearly varied greatly as did the strength of the expectation and the extent to which the time of death could be predicted. If a person had a bad accident, a sudden heart attack or stroke, his death might be expected for a short time afterwards, whereas before then it would be quite unexpected. In contrast, the death of an elderly person suffering from a chronic illness might be vaguely expected over many years. These ambiguities are illustrated by the fact that for one in ten of the so-called expected deaths the respondents later said they did not know, or only half knew, that the person was dying, while for a quarter of the deaths they described as unexpected they had known the person was unlikely to recover.

The proportion of unexpected deaths decline from 20% among those under 45 to 2% of those aged 85 or more. But even among the deaths at this older age only 70% were felt to have been expected—the remaining 28% were neither one nor the other. Half the accident deaths were unexpected, as were 16% of those from circulatory conditions, though few of those from other causes. Putting this the other way round, 78% of the unexpected deaths were from circulatory conditions, 12% from accidents, 10% from other causes. Six per cent of the deaths in hospital or institution were described as unexpected, 13% of those in people's homes and, not surprisingly, a high proportion, 50%, of those occurring in other places such as in ambulances, in the street or at work. Obviously, when only a tenth of all deaths were unexpected, most of the people who died must have been ill or frail for some time beforehand.

Restrictions

We asked a series of questions about people's restrictions.[1] Results are summarised in Table 8.

[1] Question 4: 'Before he died was —— ever completely bedridden?' IF YES: 'How long was that for?' Question 5: '(Before that) Was he confined mainly to bed?' IF YES: 'How long for?' Question 6: '(Before that) Was he at all restricted in what he could do inside the house?' IF YES: 'Would you say he was severely restricted, moderately restricted, or little restricted?' IF NO: 'Was he restricted in what he could do outside?'

TABLE 8 *Restrictions*[a]

	%
Bedridden for a year or more	3
Mainly confined to bed for a year or more	6
Either bedridden or mainly confined to bed for 6 months but less than 1 year	3
Either bedridden or mainly confined to bed for 3 months but less than 6 months	8
Severely restricted inside house for 3 months or more	17
Moderately restricted inside house for 3 months or more	15
Other restriction inside or outside for 3 months or more	14
Bedridden or mainly confined to bed for less than 3 months	15
Other restrictions for less than 3 months	3
None	16
Number of deaths (=100%)[b]	773

[a] Only the most severe restriction has been counted here—taking them in the order of priority as listed in the table.

[b] Inadequate information was obtained about the restrictions of 12 of the people who died. They have been omitted when calculating percentages. In other tables, too, some deaths have been excluded for similar reasons.

Two-thirds of the people had had some restriction for three months or longer, one in five of these being bedridden or mainly confined to bed. Examples of people described as being severely or moderately restricted inside their house were:

'He found it difficult to do much—if he walked across the room he was out of breath' (moderately restricted).

'Very feeble—just pottered about. Faulty eyesight and hard of hearing' (moderately restricted).

'When he wanted to go to the toilet I had to take him in case he had a dizzy attack' (moderately restricted).

'Chiefly mentally—couldn't speak properly—like a small child to look after. We had to do everything for him. Had been most active—helped neighbours with problems. He was always the one they came to. That's why this was even more distressing—to such an active man.' (severely restricted).

Naturally older people were more likely to have some restrictions than younger ones: a quarter of those who died when they were under 70 were said not to have had any restrictions, but only one in ten of those who were older.[1] And the proportions restricted in some way for three months or longer were 57% of those under 70, 76% of those older. Only 5% of all the deaths were of people under 65 who died unexpectedly, within twenty-four hours of an accident or being taken ill, and who had no reported restrictions.[2]

Symptoms

In addition to restrictions and disabilities most of the people who died suffered from a variety of symptoms before their death. Informants were asked whether the person who died had any of the symptoms listed in Table 9 in the last twelve months of his life, or any other symptoms he or the informant found distressing. Pain, sleeplessness, loss of appetite and trouble with breathing were the most commonly reported ones. About a third suffered from depression, mental confusion, lack of bladder control or nausea. Some of the other reported symptoms were dizziness, haemorrhage, black-outs, shaking, dribbling, double vision and bad temper.

Just over two-thirds had one or more symptoms reported as 'very distressing'[3] to the dead person and just under two-thirds had had some symptom for at least a year.

The length of time for which people had different symptoms and the proportion reported to have found them 'very distressing' are shown in Table 10. The top part of the table relates

[1] Another study found that unlimited movement decreased from 78% among those aged 60–64 to 14% among those of 85 or more. See Sheldon, J. H., *The Social Medicine of Old Age*, p. 24.

[2] A number of questions were subsequently omitted for these unexpected deaths under 65. The interviewers also omitted these questions for another 2% of deaths which appeared to them to fall into this category. Throughout the report these 2% have been included with the other 5% of unexpected deaths under 65.

[3] Question 42a: 'Do you think he found it very distressing, fairly distressing or not very distressing?'

TABLE 9 *Symptoms*[a]

	%
Pain	66
Sleeplessness	49
Lack of bladder control	32
Lack of bowel control	28
Unpleasant smell	15
Vomiting/feeling sick	30
Loss of appetite	48
Constipation	28
Bedsores	16
Mental confusion	36
Trouble with breathing	45
Depression	36
Other symptoms	25
No symptoms[a]	11
Average number of reported symptoms	4·3
Proportion with one or more symptoms reported as 'very distressing'	69%
Length of time they had had some symptom(s)	%
None	11
Less than a month	5
One month but less than 6 months	12
Six months but less than a year	9
A year or more	63
Number of deaths (=100%)[b]	785

[a] The questions about symptoms were not asked for the unexpected deaths of people under 65 with no reported restrictions. They have been included as having no symptoms.

[b] Small numbers for whom inadequate information was obtained have been omitted when the percentages were calculated.

to the people with the different symptoms, the bottom to all the people who died. Pain, sleeplessness, trouble with breathing, constipation and depression were the most persistent symptoms:

nearly half or more of the people who suffered from them had them for at least a year. Pain, trouble with breathing, vomiting and depression were also the symptoms most often felt to be very distressing. Incontinence and bedsores were also thought to have been very distressing to about half the people who suffered from them.

Pain was the most common distressing symptom and the one people were most likely to have had for a year or more. Trouble with breathing, depression and sleeplessness came next.

Some symptoms were reported as not very distressing to the person who died but had been upsetting to others.

> 'I thought the smell was horrible. She had a discharge from her breast but she kept it clean. After she died her husband said he could hardly stay in the same room, especially at night. They had the door propped open though.'

And one woman, describing how her father-in-law looked after his dying wife, said:

> 'The old man looked after the old woman while I did the housework and cooking. He used to wash her and make the bed. One day I thought there was a queer smell. I looked in the bed. It was soaking wet. She was dressed in lots of old skirts under her nightdress and the bed mattress was soaking as well. I gave her a good bath and tore an old flannelette sheet into three to make a draw sheet. We hadn't got a waterproof sheet so I put my mac. under the draw sheet.' (Loss of bowel and bladder control for three–six months reported as 'not very distressing'.)

People dying at younger ages were much more likely to suffer from vomiting or sickness and rather more likely to have pain, loss of appetite and, more surprisingly, sleeplessness,[1] than people dying at older ages. But at the older ages people more often suffered from incontinence and mental confusion. These differences are shown in Table 11.

These age variations in reported symptoms arose partly because of age differences in the cause of death. People dying from cancer were reported to have a high proportion of

[1] Among the population sleeplessness increases with age. See Dunnell, Karen and Cartwright, Ann, *Medicine Takers, Prescribers and Hoarders*, p. 112.

TABLE 10 *Length and distress of symptoms*

	Pain	*Sleeplessness*	*Loss of bladder control only*	*Loss of bowel control only*	*Loss of both bowel and bladder control*	*Unpleasant smell*	*Vomiting*	*Loss of appetite*	*Constipation*	*Bedsores*	*Mental confusion*	*Breathing trouble*	*Depression*
Length:	%	%	%	%	%	%	%	%	%	%	%	%	%
Less than a month	12	8	38	38	45	25	29	24	15	42	40	23	17
One month but less than a year	29	34	30	28	32	40	43	48	34	50	31	24	36
A year or more	59	58	32	34	23	35	28	28	51	8	29	53	47
Proportion reported as very distressing to deceased	63%	35%	50%	52%	51%	32%	56%	22%	33%	49%	27%	63%	55%
Number with symptom (=100%)	515	380	63	32	185	118	233	372	222	127	280	350	275
Proportion of all people who died:													
a) Who had symptom for a year or more	37%	27%	2%	1%	5%	5%	8%	13%	14%	1%	10%	24%	17%
b) Who found symptom very distressing	42%	17%	4%	2%	12%	5%	17%	11%	9%	8%	10%	28%	19%
Number (=100%)[a]	785												

[a] Those for whom inadequate information was obtained have been omitted when calculating the percentages.

TABLE 11 *Symptoms by age at death*

	Age at death							
	15–44	*45–54*	*55–64*	*65–69*	*70–74*	*75–79*	*80–84*	*85+*
	%	%	%	%	%	%	%	%
Pain	77	73	68	69	71	62	60	58
Sleeplessness	60	56	49	51	50	49	42	42
Loss of bladder control	26	25	26	27	32	41	30	43
Loss of bowel control	17	25	24	26	28	35	22	36
Unpleasant smell	11	20	14	14	14	20	10	19
Vomiting/feeling sick	57	45	34	29	26	22	29	19
Loss of appetite	57	55	54	44	46	48	45	39
Constipation	31	36	25	28	26	29	32	27
Bedsores	20	18	15	15	14	11	17	26
Mental confusion	31	24	25	30	41	43	39	52
Trouble with breathing	37	36	48	52	55	39	46	34
Depression	51	42	37	33	38	36	27	34
Other	29	25	24	24	24	25	23	27
None[a]	23	22	21	9	5	4	8	4
Average number	4·9	4·7	4·1	4·2	4·5	4·4	4·0	4·2
Number of deaths (=100%)	35	55	142	126	110	112	99	96

[a] The questions about symptoms were not asked about the unexpected deaths of people under 65 with no reported restrictions. They have been included as having no symptoms.

symptoms: notably pain, sleeplessness, vomiting or nausea, and loss of appetite. This can be seen from Table 12.

Apart from those dying as a result of an accident, deaths from ischaemic heart disease (coronary thrombosis) were associated with the fewest symptoms: an average of 2·9% compared with about half as many again for other forms of circulatory disease and respiratory conditions and nearly twice as many for cancer.

Seven-tenths of those who died from respiratory conditions were reported to have had trouble with breathing, and loss of bladder control was also relatively frequent for these people. Mental confusion was most common among those dying of cerebrovascular disease (stroke) and respiratory conditions—partly a reflection of their age.

So far we have shown that just over half the people who died were confined to bed or restricted inside the house in some way that informants felt was moderate or severe for at least three

TABLE 12 *Symptoms by cause of death*

	Cause of death						
	Neoplasms	*Ischaemic heart disease*	*Cerebro-vascular disease*	*Other circulatory disease*	*Respiratory conditions*	*Accidents*	*Others*
	%	%	%	%	%	%	%
Pain	87	58	57	64	55	35	69
Sleeplessness	69	37	37	47	55	25	40
Loss of bladder control	38	16	38	32	44	5	37
Loss of bowel control	37	11	34	26	35	5	27
Unpleasant smell	26	5	13	17	16	—	15
Vomiting/feeling sick	54	17	17	31	25	5	25
Loss of appetite	76	28	31	54	46	25	48
Constipation	42	19	20	31	24	10	38
Bedsores	24	4	17	21	19	5	19
Mental confusion	36	19	50	41	47	15	40
Trouble with breathing	47	41	35	55	71	10	31
Depression	45	27	33	31	40	35	37
Other	31	14	28	28	26	15	23
None[a]	2	21	8	14	4	48	12
Average number	5·9	2·9	3·8	4·5	4·7	1·8	4·3
Number of deaths (=100%)[b]	215	187	133	79	97	21	53

[a] People who died unexpectedly before they were 65 have been included as having no symptoms.
[b] Small numbers for whom inadequate information was available have been excluded when the percentages were calculated.

months before their death. Nearly two-thirds had had at least one symptom for a year or longer. Where did they live during this time and who lived with them?

Home circumstances

Nine per cent spent the whole of their last year in a hospital or institution. As expected, a high proportion of these people were very restricted: 14% had been bedridden or mainly confined to bed for a year or longer and a further 44% had been severely restricted or confined to bed for at least three months. But 32% were described as being only moderately restricted for three months or more, or having more severe restrictions for a shorter time, and 10% were said to have no restrictions at all. Most of these had been in a 'permanent residence of an institutional nature'. The matron of one of these explained:

> 'Everyone must be ambulatory who comes here. We have no one qualified to nurse the sick. Mr —— had not been ill at all or complained of anything. He used to do the shopping for others. He went out alone every day. He just collapsed while setting the tables in the dining room' (died of coronary thrombosis).

The rest of this section describes the home circumstances of the other 91%. The household composition of men and women of different ages is shown in Table 13. One in seven and nearly a quarter of those aged 85 or more lived on their own when they died or went into hospital for the last time. Over a third of the men and about a quarter of the women lived just with a wife or husband, but the proportion was lower for older people. Slightly over two-fifths of both men and women lived with people of a younger generation—nearly always their children. This proportion was highest, 85%, for the people under 45, dropped to just under a third of those aged 65–69 and then rose to half of those aged 85 or more.

People were more likely to live with married daughters than with married sons.[1] Those living with relatives of a younger generation were as likely to live with unmarried sons as

[1] See also Willmott, Peter and Young, Michael, *Family and Class in a London Suburb*, p. 72.

TABLE 13 *Variations in household composition with sex and age*[a]

	Sex		Age of deceased at death[a]								
	Men	Women	15–44	45–54	55–64	65–69	70–74	75–79	80–84	85+	All
	%	%	%	%	%	%	%	%	%	%	%
On own	10	19	—	—	9	13	14	20	24	23	14
With spouse only	37	25	3	31	41	47	39	28	15	17	31
With spouse and others of same or older generation only	2	2	—	2	4	2	2	1	—	—	2
With spouse and others of a younger generation	29	13	76	54	29	21	12	11	6	4	22
With relatives of younger generation	15	30	9	4	12	10	25	27	41	46	22
With relatives of same or older generation	4	7	9	5	4	3	5	10	5	7	6
With unrelated people only	2	3	3	4	1	3	3	2	4	—	2
In guesthouse, etc.	1	1	—	—	—	1	—	1	5	3	1
Number of deceased (=100%)[b]	388	325	34	55	139	120	104	96	93	71	713

[a] Includes one person for whom age was not known.
[b] Excluding those in hospital or institution for a year or more. It relates to their household composition at the time of their death or when they went into hospital for the last time.

TABLE 14 *Living with people of a younger generation*

	Those living with spouse as well	*Those living without spouse*	*All those living with relatives of a younger generation*
Living with:[a]	%	%	%
Married daughter	5	42	24
Married son	3	13	8
Unmarried daughter	30	22	26
Unmarried son	44	12	28
Unmarried son(s) and daughter(s)	16	1	8
Other relatives of a younger generation	2	10	6
Number living with relatives of a younger generation (=100%)	151	156	307

[a] In the classification married children took precedence over unmarried and children over other relatives.

unmarried daughters (see Table 14); but those who were widowed more often lived with unmarried daughters.

Seven per cent of people had gone to live with someone, usually their children, as they became ill or older.[1] For 5%, someone had gone to live with them.

> 'His sister came to live with him the last time he was home. After his stroke he came to us [son and daughter-in-law] and we looked after him. He kept going into hospital and seemed to improve. The hospital doctor said he could go home if someone lived with him. His sister agreed to do this. I built him a small bungalow with all the devices suitable for a semi-paralysed man—he only lived in it for four months, though.'

A quarter had made a variety of other changes in their house-

[1] Question 34: 'Were there any changes in ——'s household arrangements after he became ill/as he got older? Did anyone come to live with him? Did he go to live with anyone else?' These questions were not asked about the 7% under 65 with no reported restrictions who died unexpectedly—within twenty-four hours of an accident or being taken ill. They have been included as not making any changes because of ill health or old age.

hold arrangements. These included 'his cousin came twice a week to generally clear up', 'we used to take our meals to have with her the last five weeks', and 'used the back room downstairs as a bedroom'.

It is obviously easier for people to cope with illness and disabilities if their homes are convenient, well-equipped and with few stairs. Older people living alone, or just with others of the same or an older generation, are particularly vulnerable if their homes are difficult to run. Table 15 shows some of the housing conditions in which different sorts of people were living.

Older people had fewer amenities than younger ones and among the older people those living alone were the least well off.[1] A third of the people aged 65 or more who lived on their own had an outside lavatory. Older people were more likely to have their bedroom on the ground floor, but, associated with this, rather more of them had steps or stairs between their bedroom and the lavatory.

We asked respondents whether they thought the dead person's house or flat was very convenient, fairly convenient or rather inconvenient for them after they became ill or old. Three-fifths thought it very convenient, one in six rather inconvenient. It was expected that respondents would regard homes with an outside lavatory as less convenient than those with an inside one. It might also be reasonable for respondents to have higher standards for older people and those who lived alone than for younger ones or people living with others. But, as Table 15 shows, the proportion who felt the dead person's home was convenient did not vary in relation to their age or by whether they lived alone or not. Houses with outside lavatories were rated as rather inconvenient more often than other houses, 38% compared with 12%, but two-fifths of our respondents regarded houses with outside lavatories as very convenient for the people living in them.

When people had been restricted before they died their homes were less often described as very convenient: 58% compared with 83% for those who had not been restricted. But those who were restricted were as likely as others to live

[1] See also Buckle, Judith R., *Work and Housing of Impaired Persons in Great Britain*, pp. 79–80.

TABLE 15 *Housing conditions*[a]

	People aged 65 or more living:					
	On own	With spouse or others of same or older generation only	With others	Total	People under 65	All deaths
Lavatory:	%	%	%	%	%	%
Own indoor	59	78	78	75	86	78
Shared indoor	7	1	2	2	1	2
Outside	34	21	20	23	13	20
Bathroom:	%	%	%	%	%	%
Own with running hot and cold	58	78	84	77	89	81
Shared with running hot and cold	10	1	1	3	1	2
Neither	32	21	15	20	10	17
Proportion with bedroom at ground level	51%	48%	38%	44%	28%	30%
Proportion with no steps or stairs between bedroom and lavatory	53%	67%	67%	65%	73%	67%
Proportion who had lived in the same house for 20 years or more	48%	49%	40%	45%	35%	42%
House or flat thought to be:	%	%	%	%	%	%
Very convenient	60	62	61	61	60	61
Fairly convenient	21	23	23	23	24	23
Rather inconvenient	19	15	16	16	16	16
Number of deaths (=100%)[b]	86	178	211	475	180	655

[a] Excluding the 9% who had been in hospital or other institution for a year or more and the unexpected deaths of people under 65.
[b] Those for whom inadequate information was obtained are included in the total but have been excluded when calculating percentages.

in households with their own indoor lavatory or a bathroom with running hot and cold water.[1] The restricted seemed rather more likely to have their bedroom at ground level: 41% against 30% of those with no restrictions, but no less likely to have stairs between their bedroom and the lavatory.

Possibly one of the reasons why the homes of people living alone were as often described as 'very convenient' although they had fewer amenities was that more of those living alone were said not to have had any restrictions: 27% compared with 15% of others. But when people lived alone we were less likely to be able to interview someone in close contact with them during the last year of their lives, so our informant may have been less aware of their problems.

Help needed

Perceptions of people's need for help are also likely to vary with the knowledge and closeness of the person interviewed. The types of help the people who died were reported to need while they were at home are shown in Table 16. The 9% who were in a hospital or institution throughout the year have been omitted from the table. They may have needed help at home before they were admitted, but this was some time ago so, we did not feel it was appropriate to ask about it.

Eighteen per cent were said not to have needed help of any sort before their death. But nearly a third had needed some help with personal or self care for at least a year and just over a fifth had needed some help at night for a month or longer. Half or more of those requiring social care or assistance with housework or financial aid had needed this for over a year and between one in seven and one in five of those who needed more intensive and demanding care such as to be given bedpans or bottles or to be lifted had such long-term needs.

Those living alone were least often perceived to be needing help with nursing or night care but the ones most likely to

[1] Buckle found that the only difference in housing amenities among people with varying degrees of handicap was that a lower proportion of persons who were very handicapped or needing special care had exclusive use of hot water, fixed bath and inside W.C. She thought this was likely to be because younger people were living in better accommodation than elderly persons (op. cit., p. 80).

TABLE 16 *Types of help needed while at home*[a]

Help with self care	%
To be lifted	49
Washing or shaving	54
Getting in or out of bath	30
Dressing or undressing	42
Getting in or out of bed	44
Washing hair	37
Cutting toenails	48
Giving bedpan or bottle	24
Getting to lavatory or commode	44
None	30
Length of time needed any help with self care	%
None needed	30
Less than a week	8
A week but less than a month	10
One month but less than three months	11
Three months but less than a year	11
A year or more	30
Nursing care	%
Giving medicine or tablets	45
Injections	20
Bandaging or other dressing	15
Regular temperature-taking	5
Massaging or exercises	13
Enema	6
Other nursing procedure	10
None of these	41
Help at night with	%
Getting to lavatory	18
Bedpan	11
Medicine-taking	16
Injections or other treatment	2
Drinks	30
Company	31
Other things	10
None of these	53
Length of time needed help at night	%
None needed	53
Less than a week	14
A week but less than a month	12
One month but less than three months	8
Three months but less than a year	7
A year or more	6
Social care	%
To take him/her out	31
To read to him/her	8
To write letters for him/her	20
To collect his/her pension	50
To change his/her library books	12
None of these	39
Financial help	%
Yes	22
No	78
Help with housework[b]	%
Shopping	40
Preparing/cooking food	31
Cleaning house	39
Washing clothes	35
None of these	37

Number of deaths excluding those in hospital or institution for twelve months or more (=100%)[c] 713.

[a] These questions were not asked about the unexpected deaths of people under 65, with no reported restrictions. They have been included in the table as not needing any help at home.

[b] Includes help needed by deceased or respondent if either of them were responsible for the housework.

[c] Those for whom inadequate information was obtained have been omitted when calculating percentages.

have needed help with housework. Those living with relatives of a younger generation were more often reported to need care than those living with their spouse or others of the same or an older generation. These differences are shown in Table 17.

TABLE 17 *Household composition and help needed while at home*[a]

	On own	*With spouse or others of same or older generation*	*With relatives of younger generation*	*With unrelated people or in guest house*
Needed:	%	%	%	%
Help with self care	53	66	79	67
Nursing care	32	58	68	50
Night care	18	47	56	42
Social care	52	58	67	58
Financial help	26	18	24	21
Help with housework	78	47	50	33
None	17	20	15	25
Number of deaths (=100%)	99	274	305	24

[a] Those who had been in a hospital or other institution for a year or more before they died have been excluded. Those who died unexpectedly before they were 65 have been included as not needing any help.

If help is readily to hand it will more often be given and then be seen to be needed. If it is not available people will often manage without it and may therefore be thought not to need it. Sometimes having to do things for themselves may keep those living alone more active and free from restrictions.[1] But it would also seem that at certain stages of difficulty some people go to live with relatives.

Sources of care

Who gave help when it was needed? Few people were said not to get any help when they needed it, but respondents may

[1] Another study found that elderly people living alone or with a spouse were no less likely than elderly people living with others to report various symptoms but were more likely to go out. See Lance, Hilary, *Transport Services in General Practice*, pp. 46–7.

not always have been aware of un-met needs. When people are helped at least the person who helps knows about it, and of course some may have been helped when they could have managed on their own if necessary. The threshold of need is often difficult to define and in practice is likely to have been determined in part by the help available.

Table 18 shows that wives, husbands and daughters were the people most likely to help with nearly all types of care.[1] (The one exception was financial problems. This is discussed in Chapter 7.)

TABLE 18 *Help with different types of care while at home*

	Self care	*Nursing care*	*Help at night*	*Social care*	*Financial care*	*House-work*	*All types of care*
	%	%	%	%	%	%	%
Spouse	46	32	53	36	—	20	37
Daughter	31	22	31	34	11	31	30
Son	12	4	16	14	16	9	11
Brother/sister	6	4	6	7	1	5	6
Other relative	20	11	22	18	9	23	19
Friend or neighbour	7	4	11	12	—	18	10
District nurse	19	35	3	—	—	—	15
Home help, hairdresser or chiropodist	4	1	—	1	—	13	4
Other professional or voluntary help	3	15	6	3	66	7	7
No one	1	2	—	2	15	9	3
Number of different types of help needed (=100%)[a]	2,608	796	453	838	140	1,008	5,843

[a] The percentages add to more than 100 as some people had help from more than one sort of person.

Relatives, friends and neighbours gave nearly all the social care and help at night, most of the help with housework and

[1] Similar findings are reported by Hinton: 'Nursing usually falls to the wife when the man is ill and the daughter when the woman is sick.' Hinton, John, *Dying*, p. 149.

self care and much of the nursing care. The district nurse helped with a third of the nursing needs and a fifth of the self care problems. Home helps were a source of aid for one-in-eight of the housework needs.

The proportions of *people* who died who had help from nurses, home helps and other local authority and voluntary sources is shown in Table 19 for those who were at home for some time during the year before they died.

TABLE 19 *Help from nurses, home helps and other local authority and voluntary sources*

	%
District nurse	33
Health visitor	8
Other nurse	5
Home help	10
Special laundry service	2
Chiropodist	11
Vicar, priest, minister or other church worker	29
Other local authority or voluntary service	12
None of these[a]	41
Number of deaths excluding those in hospital or institution for a year or more (=100%)	703

[a] Those who died unexpectedly have been included as not having any help.

A third had been helped by a district nurse, one in ten by a home help. A study in part of Glasgow of deaths among people aged 65 and over found fewer, 13%, helped by a district nurse; a similar proportion, 11%, by a home help.[1] Three-tenths of those in the present survey had been visited by a vicar, priest, minister or other church worker.

But the professional person most likely to have visited the person who died in the year before his death was the general practitioner. Eighty-eight per cent had had a home visit from him and all but 4% had had some contact with a general practitioner during that time.

In addition many received some care from the hospital. As

[1] Isaacs, Bernard *et al.*, 'The concept of pre-death'.

well as the 9% who spent at least twelve months before they died in a hospital or institution, 61% were in hospital for some time during the last year of their lives, leaving 30% who were never in-patients in that time. A quarter of this last group had some contact with the hospital at out-patient departments, so all but 22% of the people who died had some hospital or institutional care in the last twelve months of their lives. Another study of 2,243 deaths between ages 15 and 74 showed that 26% of the people who died had not been referred to hospital for investigation or treatment: a proportion the author found 'surprisingly high'.[1]

Summary

Few people die completely unexpectedly with no previous illness. For most the last year of their lives is a time when they are restricted, suffer from a variety of unpleasant symptoms and need help to enable them to cope with their disabilities. All but 9% spent at least some of their last year at home; most of them lived with relatives but one in seven lived alone. A quarter of those aged 85 or more lived alone, and half of them shared a home with one of their children.

Help and support came from a variety of sources: relatives, friends, neighbours, district nurses, home helps, ministers of religion, general practitioners and the hospital. Later chapters examine these various sources of help in more detail.

[1] Alderson, M. R., 'Referral to hospital among a representative sample of adults who died'.

3

THE EXPERIENCES OF SOME PEOPLE WITH PARTICULAR NEEDS

So far people's needs and care during the last year of their lives have been described in a general way and largely in statistical terms. This chapter focuses in more depth on people likely to have particular needs: elderly people living alone, those who had been in a hospital or institution for a year or more before they died, the bedridden, the mentally confused and those who died when they were young (under 45).

Elderly people living alone[1]

Among those aged 65 or more, the proportion of people living alone before they died or went into hospital for the last time increased with age from one in eight of those aged 65–69 to almost one in four of those aged 80 or more. Women, the widowed, the single and the childless were relatively likely to live alone.[2] This is shown in Table 20.

Tunstall found that most of the old people living alone preferred it that way: 'the popular preference, given reasonable health, is to maintain regular contact with children, siblings, or others—without imposing upon them, or becoming too dependent on them'.[3] Although we do not know what the people in our study really felt, those living alone were reported to have had fewer symptoms than those living with others: an average of 3·7 compared with 4·5. And, as we saw earlier, those living alone had fewer restrictions: among the elderly 28% of

[1] This section is based on those who died when they were 65 or more. Those who had been in a hospital or institution for a year or more before they died have been excluded.

[2] Similar findings were reported by Tunstall, Jeremy, *Old and Alone*, pp. 47–53.

[3] Tunstall, op. cit., p. 56. See also Townsend, Peter, and Wedderburn, Dorothy, *The Aged in the Welfare State*, p. 66; they found that 91% of the old people in their sample who lived alone preferred to continue doing so.

TABLE 20 *Old people living alone*

	Proportion living alone					
	Men		Women		Both sexes	
Age						
65–69	11%	(75)	18%	(45)	13%	(120)
70–74	13%	(60)	16%	(44)	14%	(104)
75–79	15%	(41)	24%	(55)	20%	(96)
80–84	16%	(38)	29%	(55)	24%	(93)
85+	21%	(24)	23%	(47)	23%	(71)
Marital status						
Single	33%[a]	(15)	29%	(31)	30%	(46)
Married	1%	(145)	0%	(67)	0%	(212)
Widowed, divorced or separated	34%	(73)	32%	(142)	32%	(215)
Living children						
None	25%	(45)	34%	(59)	30%	(104)
One	9%	(53)	18%	(60)	14%	(113)
Two	14%	(50)	22%	(40)	18%	(90)
Three	3%	(33)	6%	(33)	5%	(66)
Four or more	16%	(43)	20%	(45)	18%	(88)
Son(s) only	12%	(41)	21%	(38)	16%	(79)
Daughter(s) only	10%	(48)	14%	(57)	12%	(105)
Son(s) and daughter(s)	11%	(91)	18%	(82)	14%	(173)
All those aged 65 or more	14%	(238)	22%	(246)	18%	(484)

The figures in brackets are the numbers on which the percentages are based (=100%). Those in a hospital or other institution for a year or more before they died have not been included.
[a] Based on less than 20 cases.

those living alone and 11% of those living with others had no restrictions. But again these differences may be partly due to the perceptions of our respondents and the taciturnity of those choosing to live alone. Symptoms they were apparently less likely to have suffered from were sleeplessness (39% against 51%), loss of appetite (29% against 52%), vomiting (17% against 29%), bedsores (6% against 19%) and trouble with breathing (33% against 52%). However, there was one symptom which was reported more often for those living alone. This was depression: 46% of those living alone compared with 32% of other elderly people were said to have been depressed.[1]

In the previous chapter we saw that people living alone were seen as less likely to have needed nursing care, help with self care and help at night than those living with others. They were felt to have been as often in need of financial help and as more likely to have needed help with housework.

These differences in need were reflected in the help received from various professional helpers (Table 21); but again there is the danger that need is not perceived, particularly by people outside the household, until some help is given. Those living on their own were much more likely to have had a home help but less likely to have been helped by a district nurse. There was a suggestion that health visitors were more likely to visit old people living on their own than those living with others.

TABLE 21 *Help from various professionals*

	People aged 65 or more		
	Living alone	*Living with others*	*All aged 65 or more*
	%	%	%
District nurse	24	41	38
Health visitor	15	9	10
Other nurse	1	7	6
Home help	35	7	12
Special laundry service	—	1	1
Chiropodist	20	15	16
Vicar, priest, or other church worker	26	34	33
Other official or voluntary worker	15	12	13
No official or voluntary worker	33	31	32
Number of deaths (=100%)	85	385	470

[1] Somewhat similar findings are reported in Goldberg, E. M. *et al.*, *Helping the Aged*, p. 70.

Church workers, on the other hand, were rather less likely to visit those living alone.

Although those living alone were said to have fewer symptoms than elderly people living with others, they were less likely to have died in their own home: 30% compared with 50%. And those living alone spent more of the last year of their lives in a hospital or institution: 24% were there for between three and twelve months compared with 7% of those living with others. Once people living alone are admitted to hospital they are less likely to be discharged to die at home within a year. Only 7% of those living alone had been in hospital during the last year of their lives but did not die there compared with 20% of those living with others.

Hospitals and institutions were obviously caring for people who would have been looked after at home if they had lived with relatives or friends. But old people living alone may be deeply attached to their homes and reluctant to leave them even though their ill health makes it difficult for them to be looked after there.

> A widow of 72 whose husband died between two and five years earlier had lived in the same house for over twenty years. She'd had depression and trouble with breathing for over a year before she died. She did not want to go to hospital and her married daughter who had looked after her explained, 'she had such a dread of hospitals—which may have developed because my father died there—I hoped I'd never have to persuade her to go'. But she had died at home from a coronary thrombosis.

> 'The doctor wanted him in hospital but he wouldn't go. He even got a bed for him. I stood and looked at him—he said "What are you staring at me for?" I said "I'm thinking what a lot they could do for you in hospital." He said "So you're one of them—just thinking how soon you can get me out of my own house. Well, I'm not going." The ambulance was due to come the next morning but he died during the night' (neighbour about a widowed man of 83).

Altogether twenty-six old people who lived alone had died at home. Two of them had been confined mainly to bed for six months or longer.

> One, a woman in her seventies, had had a stroke. Her son explained: 'When she was first confined to bed we'd each take her for a weekend. There's six of us—two brothers and four sisters—but by the time she'd been round us all once, she'd had enough—didn't want to move around.' They'd worked out a rota sytem—all the sons and daughters and one daughter-in-law, so it was once a week. Whoever was to stay at night bathed her and gave her breakfast. One son, the respondent, worked fairly near his mother's house and went round four times during the day, missing his tea and coffee breaks. Also, if she was in need, a neighbour would ring him at work and he would go round—often to put her on the commode as she wouldn't let anyone outside the family help her with this.

> The other was a woman in her eighties who'd had cancer for eleven years. Her daughter told us how her own daughter, the woman's granddaughter, used to call in on her way home and then go back for the night. The granddaughter had slept on the settee for two years.

Both people had some help from a district nurse—the first for between one and three months, the second for less than a week. The relatives said they would have liked more help from her.

Another single man was described as having been severely restricted for more than a year. He had arthritis and diabetes.

> 'He couldn't bend at all—could hardly walk his legs were so swollen and his toes were rotten—I used to dress them.' This was said by the home help who had known him for between two and five years and described herself as a close friend. 'I used to go two hours a day seven days a week.' He'd also been helped by a male friend to get in and out of the bath, by a cousin who took him out sometimes and by a district nurse for about a month. The home help thought the district nurse 'should have come every day to do his feet' and would have liked her to help 'clean him up'. He had been doubly incontinent for over six months. From her point of view she felt it would have been better for

> him to be in hospital. 'He needed a lot of looking after' but 'he didn't like hospitals—said he was caged in. His death [in August] upset me. You see I gave him up after Christmas—it was too heavy for me. I was shocked when I heard. I'm sure he missed me. He had several since me—they won't stick it you see.'

None of the others were said to have been so restricted. A third of those dying at home were said not to have had any restrictions.

> A man of 84 was said by his landlord never to be ill—'He lived at the top of two flights and was never even out of breath. I woke up in the morning at 5.30. I didn't see him the night before and for some reason I felt uneasy about him but there was no reason. It so happens that another person living in rooms here heard a bump about 8.30 the previous night but thought nothing of it. About nine of the morning I got my nephew to go up and see if the old man was all right and he found him dead on the floor' (cause of death on the death certificate given as purulent bronchitis and old age).

> 'She'd had a very bad cold but it was getting better. I went away on the Saturday and she wasn't well but she sent my husband [the dead person's husband's brother] home and said she'd have a nice sleep. But in the morning the blinds weren't drawn and the milk was still out so they broke in and she was dead' (woman of 78 who died of pneumonia).

> A man of 67 died of coronary thrombosis. 'He had an attack [coronary thrombosis] and died within fifteen minutes.' A friend who 'saw him two or three times most days' was with him when he had the attack and stayed with him until he died. 'The doctor came too late but said there was nothing he could have done.'

> A man described how his mother 'was found dead in bed in the morning as if asleep. Her little radio was still playing' (died 'suddenly from a thrombosis' aged 69).

The hazards of living alone are illustrated by the death of one woman of 81.

There was a coroner's report and her daughter explained:

> 'Apparently she was filling her hot water bottle at night when she collapsed. When found the kettle was on the floor, the bottle in her hand and the house filled with gas. The coroner was unable to say if she'd died from a coronary or just collapsed from it and the death was brought on by gas fumes. The verdict? An accident. She was an active woman before this with no previous restriction apart from general old age, deafness, loss of sight in one eye and loss of memory. The doctor said at the inquest she was a very fit woman for her age'.

These brief case histories about the deaths of people aged 65 or more who lived alone reveal wide variations in the social and medical circumstances of death. There are those who died suddenly with little or no warning; but among these were some whose end was peaceful, others whose 'sudden' death may have been preceded by hours of loneliness, fear, pain and helplessness. Those living alone, at any age, are inevitably exposed to the risk of this type of death. Such hazards have to be set beside the privacy, independence and pleasures that many derive from living alone. But although not all the risks can be eliminated they can be reduced, and there are many ways of improving communications and eliminating potential home hazards which could help those who are particularly exposed.[1]

At the other extreme, a number of those dying in hospital or institution, and some dying at home although they lived alone, had suffered from various restrictions and symptoms for a long time. Some were reluctant to leave their homes and go to places where their care could be arranged more easily. They might be less reluctant if the residential institutions and homes for the aged were more attractive places.[2] Data from this survey show that the care given by relatives and friends and supplemented by neighbours and community services, although often extensive, is frequently insufficient to meet the needs of the elderly infirm.

[1] See Brandon, Ruth, *Seventy Plus*, pp. 59–78.

[2] See Townsend, Peter, *The Last Refuge*, for a description of such places in 1959.

The institutionalised

Seventy-two of the people who died were reported to have been in a hospital or some other institution for over a year before they died. A quarter of them had been there for one to two years, two-fifths for two to five years and a third for five years or more. The dying person's increasing needs for nursing care were often cited as a reason for his entering an institution.

> 'He'd got very feeble after my mother died, and was blind. He couldn't look after himself. After my mother died I went down to see him each day but it was too much so he went in the home for old people.' (He was in the old people's home for over five years, was transferred to hospital and lived there for three days before dying of 'old age' according to his daughter.)

Increasing disability and incontinence were the main reasons for the hospitalisation of one 77-year-old woman. She had a very convenient ground-floor flat where she lived on her own. Her nephew and his wife (our informant) lived upstairs and were mainly responsible for looking after her. She had been bedridden for about a year before going into hospital. She was deaf, suffered from arthritis, weighed fourteen stone and was doubly incontinent. It was the need to change the soiled bed continually that led to her hospitalisation.

> 'The G.P. got her into hospital, it was impossible. It was necessary for her. It's so much easier for two nurses who are trained. He came one day when I was trying to clean up the bed—she'd just soiled it. He said, "You can't go on like this. I'll get her into hospital". I just didn't feel anything [about her dying in hospital], I was exhausted. She was deaf—we got her a deaf-aid but she wouldn't use it. She was so cut off—it was terrible really. She was in hospital for the last year. When she was at home it meant changing the bed twice a day. Sometimes I think she enjoyed it. She used to look at me and say, "I've wet the bed". She seemed almost pleased. It was a terrible job. I wouldn't mind washing sheets once a week but washing blankets every day was a different thing. She wanted to

come home but I just couldn't manage. It took two of them to lift her. I thought I might have managed but I was working in the business, looking after my daughter and I just couldn't manage. When it comes to washing four or five blankets every day it is too much. My husband said I mustn't have her back, it was too much.'

So she remained in hospital until she died of pneumonia.

Sometimes a change in the home circumstances made it impossible to care for the sick person any longer. The matron of an old people's home gave the death of a resident's sisters as the reason for her going to the home: 'She lived alone. Her sisters had died, that is why she came to us.'

Another woman, whose 90-year-old aunt died in hospital told how a combination of her aunt's and uncle's increasing age and infirmity and their awkward home conditions resulted in their being admitted to hospital. They had lived on their own in a first floor flat.

> 'It was a nice little flat. They were very comfortable there except for the stairs. Uncle could manage them, he used to go out on his own . . . but it was the stairs down to the front door that she couldn't manage. She probably could have got down them, but she was afraid to, so she didn't go out. She and uncle were admitted to hospital because of their age, more on her account. She could be very trying and it was more than uncle could stand. She kept on turning things out, turning drawers out and cleaning out cupboards. Uncle liked a bit of peace but he didn't get it. She didn't want to go into hospital at all, but uncle just couldn't stand it. But she seemed to get worse quickly when they took her in.' And there she died of a cerebral haemorrhage.

Once they went into an institution, how far were the people who died isolated from their relatives and friends? The long-term patients were likely to have had fewer visitors than other people who had been in hospital. Those in hospital or an institution for the whole year had an average of 4·8 visitors, compared with 6·8 for those in hospital for a shorter time. Part of the reason for this is that comparatively few of those in hospital or other institution for a year or more were married

(10% compared with 57%) and husband and wives were the most assiduous visitors.[1]

For people in institutions visitors are one of the few links with the outside world. Being able to talk to relatives and friends from outside helps to maintain people's self-identity.[2]

One man whose mother died in an old people's home used to visit the other old people there when he went to see his mother. His wife told the story.

> 'After she died, the matron said, "Don't stop coming, the old people will miss you." My husband went once, but it upset him so much to see someone else sitting in his mother's chair that he couldn't go again.'

Some of the respondents were critical of relatives who did not visit.

> 'This road is full of our relatives—every house but one. And not one of them ever went to see my Dad. I'll never forgive them for that.' (The hospital was 30 minutes' journey away.)

Mental hospitals and psychiatric institutions still seem to have a stigma attached to them which frightens off visitors.

> 'The majority have no visitors. People handy but don't go because it's a mental hospital.'

> 'I think his family forgot him years before he came here [home for subnormals]. Very common to all these chaps. The first two months relatives can't keep off doorstep, then they disappear, lose contact completely—move without telling you.'

Instances like the following were uncommon.

> A 77-year-old woman had been admitted to a home about two years before her death. Her daughter, our respondent, visited her regularly and 'she came to spend every weekend at our house—she was able to get about. She enjoyed the

[1] Question 16(b): 'Who visited —— most often?'

[2] See Goffman, Erving, *Asylums*, for a more detailed account of the erosion of self-identity which can take place when people enter institutions.

change every weekend'. She was transferred to hospital for an operation two weeks before she died.

For most of the people who spent the whole of their last year in hospitals or other institutions, contact with relatives and friends was confined to their visits. The staff and inmates of the institution were their constant companions, but they were involuntary companions thrown together by processes over which they had little or no control. Townsend in his study of residential institutions for the elderly found that less than a fifth of the new residents in the homes he was studying had a friend among the other residents.[1] Some of the people who had been in hospitals or institutions for some time seemed to have adjusted to the life there and had had time to get to know the staff.

> 'The nurses were marvellous to her. She had times when she would be laughing and noisier. Then she'd cheek the nurses and they liked it. They used to tease her and make a fuss of her. They loved her, you could see the way they looked after the patients and combed their hair that they really loved them.'

Many of our informants had nothing but praise for the care their relatives received while in hospital or institution. Seven out of ten of the friends and relatives made comments indicating that they were pleased with the way the person was looked after.[2] This is how one woman described the care given to her 91-year-old mother during the five years spent in hospital before she died.

> 'In the ward where mother was we were thrilled with it. They were very attentive and in the intensive care unit they were marvellous. We were very satisfied. Anyone who says anything against —— [hospital] I wouldn't believe. We were very surprised to find the nurses cared so much. The staff were really upset when she died. It was nothing strange at that hospital to see a nurse in tears after losing a patient she was fond of.'

Fourteen per cent had some grievance or expressed some

[1] Townsend, op. cit., p. 348.
[2] Those informants who were staff in an institution have been excluded.

doubts about the institution and the remaining 17% were upset or displeased with the care given to the person in one institution, but were happier with the way he was treated in another. In the following discussion we have emphasised the negative comments because they reveal the inadequacies. We hope that by drawing attention to these more staff and resources may be concentrated on those needing long-term nursing care.

A few informants described the lack of activity which is sometimes a feature of institutional life.

> 'They were short of staff and sometimes left them when they wanted to go to the toilet. It was beautifully kept and clean and had television. They had nothing to do when we were visiting but they might not have wanted to do anything anyway. There was nothing more that could have been done for auntie but I thought some of the old ladies could have been occupied. Perhaps they were when we weren't there.'

> 'That hospital should be burnt down. Herd of young and old men waiting to die. My dad used to get up at six, breakfast at seven, then they just sat and looked at each other all day—why?'

From such descriptions it is possible to see how people may react by withdrawing into isolation.[1] With nothing to look forward to except their next meal, a change into clean and dry clothing or bedding and the next visiting period, the management of their everyday life could seem out of their hands, taken over by the institution. This might lead to withdrawal, lack of awareness and concentration and even loss of control of bodily functions and mental confusion. Occasionally respondents reported that their relatives had become selfish or ill-tempered since they went into the institution and this in turn affected their relationships with those caring for them and visiting them, giving rise to further isolation. The process was sometimes exacerbated by the patient being blind, deaf or severely incapacitated in other ways. From the relatives' reports it seemed that a few of the institutions were rather like the 'total institution' outlined by Goffmann.[2]

[1] See also Townsend, op. cit., p. 105.

[2] Goffmann, op. cit., pp. 24–51.

A number of the people we interviewed were critical of institutional life because of the effect it had of cutting off entirely what were considered to be essential features of life.

> 'There was a big range of ages. They all slept together and they were all in one big day room. There wasn't room for some to do one thing and others to sit quiet. They were all mixed up together. If they could have had smaller units it would have been better, but the hospital found it difficult to get staff.'

One matron of a home for the blind told how she made a great exception for one man and allowed him a small piece of personal freedom which many would not dream of being deprived of—being allowed to smoke.

> 'He loved the fresh air—he'd been a farm labourer—and he liked his pipe, so I used to let him smoke in bed. Though it's against the rules because of insurance.'

Other criticisms of the institutions, and expressions of distress at the existence the dying people led in them, concerned the care they got, or lack of it, the food, ward conditions, the incontinence and mentally confused state of other inmates. A woman described two visits she made to her mother:

> 'I found my mother sitting out of bed in an uncomfortable canvas chair, by a window; the room icy cold, she had no heating or hot water bottle and she was in a most distressed condition. Some cold curry or mince had been served, which she could not eat. I searched for help but there was no one in authority to be found, so I gave her the attention she badly needed and got her into bed. I then left at once to make suitable arrangements for her removal.
>
> Two days later my brother and I called to collect her and found her in a soiled bed, and as before, in a cold room. The temperature in the corridor outside was 53°F. and felt considerably warmer than the room.'

Another woman was upset by the care her mother-in-law received in the chronic ward of a hospital.

> 'She was fine in the acute ward but when they moved her to

the chronic ward it was terrible. They didn't bother. They were short of staff and she was wet and bedsore. I'll never forget it. You'd better be dead than old!'

Similar feelings were expressed by the next respondent about the attention given to her father in one hospital.

> 'One time I visited him, he was filthy—could hardly speak or breathe. I went to see about it. "Oh, Matron's not in, not till 3." You just couldn't get anything done for them. A doctor was not available in hospital and the S.R.N.s just put everything down to old age. Friday before he died, took ill. My sister went to visit. "Can't see you, I'm ill." She went to get attendant. Attendant said, "Nothing wrong with him—they play up", and didn't do anything for him.'

The conditions in a mental hospital upset one man's sister.

> 'I truly believe they don't get the medical attention they should do. I know he was aggressive and though he was little he made a lot of trouble. They moved him around, each time it was worse. Last time we went—men crawling along the floor, undoing their trousers wanting to go to the toilet. A thing in the corner in a cot making an awful noise—you couldn't call it anything—I never dared look at it.'

One woman was glad that her grandmother had been moved to another hospital before she died. She thought that they were very lax in the first hospital, 'especially in geriatrics'.

> 'I was upset—we took food in to all the old folk and they absolutely fell on it. And they weren't looked after—no one had taken them to the toilet before visiting. It's awful to see an old woman squatting down to relieve herself—and they did—and none of them had special pants.'

This was distressing enough to the people visiting institutions, but those in the institution had to put up with these situations all the time; and they could be very upset by them.

> 'She was talking about other old ladies in the ward. She thought they were all people she'd known in the past. It

upset her because they used to wet the floor while they were sitting out in chairs.'

In this description we have stressed the deficiences of care and some of the unfortunate, but not necessarily inevitable, consequences of institutional life. But the majority of people we interviewed seemed pleased with the way their relatives had been cared for.

The bedridden

So far we have been concerned with people with contrasting experiences of dependence and independence: those spending all their last year in a hospital or institution, and those living alone at home. We turn now to look at two groups who are more typical in the sense that much of their care devolved on relatives living with them: the bedridden and the mentally confused. Just over half the people who died had been bedridden for some time before they died. About a third were bedridden for less than a month, just over a fifth for longer.

Slightly fewer men than women had been bedridden, 49% and 56% respectively.[1] People who died of cancer were most likely to have been bedridden for some time, and those who died of ischaemic heart disease, least likely. The length of time they were bedridden and the cause of death is shown in Table 22.

Rather more of those who died in a hospital or institution than of those who died in their own homes had been bedridden (59% compared with 48%). Even so, over a third of those who had been bedridden for three months or longer died at home. Others became bedridden before they were admitted to hospital. Thus much of the care given to bedridden patients was at home.

Becoming bedridden was often the last stage in a gradually deteriorating condition. About a third of the bedridden had been confined mainly to bed before they became completely bedridden, and three-fifths had been restricted in what they

[1] This difference persists when the age at death is standardised. It may be due to higher incidences among women of conditions such as arthritis which limit their mobility. Other studies have also found similar differences between men and women. See, for example, Hobson, W., and Pemberton, J., *The Health of the Elderly at Home*, p. 141.

TABLE 22 *Cause of death and length of time bedridden*

	Cause of death						
	Neo-plasms	*Ischaemic heart disease*	*Cerebro-vascular disease*	*Other circula-tory*	*Respir-atory*	*Other causes*	*All causes*
Length of time bedridden:	%	%	%	%	%	%	%
Not at all	28	77	40	45	42	50	47
Less than a week	14	7	14	9	14	7	11
1 week but less than 1 month	27	9	22	23	23	18	20
1 month but less than 3 months	20	4	12	14	10	5	12
3 months but less than 6 months	7	1	5	9	3	8	5
6 months or more	4	2	7	—	8	12	5
All deaths (=100%)	214	186	133	78	97	74	782

could do inside the house. But a minority of about one in eight of those who had been bedridden for some time before they died had not been restricted in any other way before they became bedridden. Of these, half were said to have been in good health before that.[1] For example, an 81-year-old woman was said to have been in good health before an accident. After that she was taken to hospital and remained there completely bedridden for eighteen weeks until she died.

> (Before accident) 'She got up at 5.30 every Monday to do washing. Did my baking—active as a 60-year-old. You name it, she did it.' (then) 'She was knocked down in November. She seemed to recover so well we thought she was going to survive, then found her injuries were so severe only her constitution made her last so long. For about three weeks before she died I knew there was not much hope.'

An 85-year-old man was in 'fair' health and had no restrictions:

> 'For his age he managed to get out and about fairly well.' Until between one and three months before his death, when

[1] Question 6: 'Would you describe his health in the last twelve months as: good, fair, poor, very poor?'

'he was very old and took to his bed. Just did not want to get up or do anything.' He was said to have died of old age.

However, the lives of most of the bedridden had been increasingly restricted physically in the years before their death. Occasionally people were kept in bed because it was easier to look after them there. A widow living with her two sons was almost solely responsible for the care of her 78-year-old mother. She told of her mother's increasing incapacity:

> 'She used to live across the road but after her first [heart] attack, I brought her over here—I thought it would be easier than going across and back all the time. She had trouble with her toe. It was black and she went into hospital and when she came home she was never the same. She often said she wished she was with her husband. That was three years before she died. She never did much but sit about. I found it such hard work getting her upstairs, I left her in bed upstairs for a day or two as I thought until my shoulder was better and she never came down again.' (She was bedridden for three to six months before she finally died of 'heart failure'.)

When people become bedridden they are no longer able to carry out their normal everyday tasks without some assistance. As Townsend pointed out in an earlier study, they may be reluctant to let other people help, even though they are not able to manage on their own, or they may let their spouse and no one else do all the work that is involved.[1] One of the nurses in our study said that this was quite common:

> 'We're coming across it all the time—where a wife has been looking after the husband until she's almost ready to go into hospital herself—she's a wreck. With a lot of old people they are very independent. They don't realise how much strain it is on the spouse.'

One man would let no one but his wife do anything for him. He had been sent home from hospital over six months before his death after an operation for cancer which 'took nearly all

[1] Townsend, Peter, *The Family Life of Old People*, pp. 56–8; Goldberg, E. M. *et al.*, *Helping the Aged*, pp. 122–3.

his stomach away'. He had been bedridden for between one and three months. He and his wife, our informant, lived with a daughter. As he became more ill and was bedridden they 'got rid of their three-piece suite and made the sitting room into a bedroom. They had a gas fire installed so that smoke wouldn't bother him.' He was doubly incontinent. This upset him very much and was a source of strain for his wife: 'The doctor said, "you can manage".' But there was a lot of work to do washing soiled bed linen: 'I used to be ill myself after it. Just used to get one lot done and there would be another lot.' He needed help with self care, such as lifting, washing and so on, as well as nursing, and help at night. His wife did everything that he needed on her own, except for taking him out. The daughter living with them and a son helped occasionally with the housework and shopping. The other daughter and four sons visited often but were not allowed to help.

> 'My husband had all the help he needed but I could have done with help for shopping and cleaning. No one [else helped with his personal care], because he wouldn't let anyone else do anything. Sometimes someone would say "What a lot of work your wife has on". But he said "That's her duty." That's how he felt about things. I didn't ask for help because I didn't want to upset my husband in any way.'

Although she was 'pleased that he died at home', there was a point when his care became too demanding and she would rather have had him back in hospital:

> 'From my point of view—about a month before he died—when he was very demanding, I would have preferred him to be in hospital. I got all the boys together one night and I told them I couldn't do for their dad any more—I was worn out, and they said, "We understand". But I did.'

She had to, for when she approached the doctor about getting her husband back into hospital: 'He said, "We can't—he's too far gone".' So that when he eventually died 'it was a happy release, I must tell you. My feet and legs were really bad.'

It may have been a 'happy release', but it was still upsetting. She had been to see her doctor 'every Tuesday for two months' because she could not sleep and had to get tablets to help her relax. She connected this with her bereavement. From her experience she had formed definite views on terminal care:

> 'I think that when people are ill and getting old and are difficult to deal with it would be good if there was some special unit in hospital where they could go. It used to worry me terrible keeping the place fresh. I used to worry about the carpet on the floor and germs. I didn't worry about myself but I used to worry about Sylvia [her daughter].'

Many people had to move furniture around or alter their rooms to make it easier to look after the dying person. One of the most commonly reported changes was to move a bed from an upstairs bedroom to a downstairs living room so that the person was nearer at hand and could see visitors more easily. Just over two-fifths of those living with bedridden people said that the rooms were altered or furniture moved round.

> 'He was exhausted when he came home. I made him a bed downstairs—the bedcovering was really nice. I made it possible for him to look nice for visitors and that. We always used to have our meals in the front room before he was ill, then we had them outside, but my hubby [who died] asked why we did this so we came back and had meals in the front room until a few days before he died.'

> 'We cleared the front parlour and brought her bed down. She didn't like it at first but she soon got used to it. I was only too pleased [to do it], it was easier for me and more people dropped in to see her. I wasn't up and down stairs so much.'

The intensity of care needed by people who were bedridden for long periods—83% of those bedridden for three months or more needed to be lifted—meant they were relatively unlikely to get all the help needed. Two-fifths of those bedridden for three months or longer were said to have needed some help or more help with personal care than they got. Sometimes inadequacy of care may have caused or aggravated some symptoms such as incontinence, constipation and bedsores. One cause of incontinence was being unable to go to the lavatory when they wanted.

A third of the people who died at home and had been bedridden at all suffered from bedsores, compared with a fifth of those dying in hospital. The proportion increased with the length of time they had been bedridden. It rose from 10% of those bedridden for less than a week to 63% of those bedridden for three months or more dying at home and 45% of those bedridden three months or more who died in hospital.

Another problem, less serious perhaps but also a distressing one, was reported by some relatives—they had trouble with the patient slipping down the bed.

> 'A hoist [would have been helpful], he kept slipping down the bed and couldn't lift himself up.'

Some relatives had to keep an eye on the bedridden person to make sure she did not try to get out of bed, especially at night.

> 'Many and many a night I sat with her until 4 a.m. because I was afraid she'd try to get out of bed and fall.'

District nurses helped many of the people who were bedridden at home. Over three-quarters of those who died at home and had been bedridden for a month or more had been visited by a district nurse. Even so the burden of care required by bedridden people was very demanding on their relatives. Two-thirds of the relatives living with people who had been bedridden for three months or more and died at home said that looking after them had restricted their own social lives. Fewer of the relatives of not so severely restricted people said this.

> 'Tied completely. Had no holiday for five years. Couldn't go away for weekends.' (A daughter who bore the brunt of looking after her 83-year-old father, bedridden for over three months.)

> 'You couldn't go out, see, and leave her. Someone had to be in all the time.' (Daughter who bore the brunt of looking after her 85-year-old mother who had been bedridden for two years.)

> 'I was tied. He wouldn't let anyone else do anything.' (This man's wife bore the brunt of looking after him. He was bedridden for more than a year.)

It seems that there is a need for more help in looking after people who are bedridden at home. Many of those who are bedridden at home have to be transferred to hospital because of the heavy demands which their relatives are unable to meet, or when there are no relatives to meet these demands. Even when a district nurse visits she may find it difficult to lift a heavy patient from the bed on to a commode when the only other available helper is a frail, old spouse. The most common type of help that people needed but did not get was help which could have been called for at any time, throughout the day or night. Of those bedridden for three months or longer two-fifths did not get enough personal help, a fifth did not get enough help at night. Relatives were responsible for most of the work involved at home, and they needed more help and advice in looking after their ill or old people. Isaacs has argued that 'The prolonged survival of many severely disabled and ill people into advanced old age is a new phenomenon in our society and has created unprecedented strain on our family and social system.'[1] Our data illustrate the problem.

The mentally confused

A third of the people who died were said to have been mentally confused at some time in the year before their death. Their confusion took a variety of forms:

> 'After the fall in February he used to have fits of giggling. I used to tell him to stop it but he'd say, "Leave me alone, I can't help it".' (A 71-year-old man who died of a stroke.)
>
> 'She went into hospital. She was very confused, she didn't know anyone except me and K. She thought all sorts of people were her family or old neighbours.' (A 76-year-old woman said to have died of 'gangrene from a broken leg'.)
>
> 'At the old people's home [he was] quite convinced they were a special regiment, visiting royalty were coming to inspect the grounds and hall and everything had to be ship-shape and they were to protect them.' (This 80-year-old man died in the old people's home of a cerebral thrombosis.)

[1] Isaacs, Bernard, 'Geriatric patients: do their families care?'

Two-fifths had become mentally confused only in the month before they died. Sometimes the confusion may have been caused by drugs given to relieve their pain or other symptoms. For example, one 74-year-old man who died of lung cancer had been mentally confused for less than a week. His doctor was said to have been unable to do anything for this, since 'injections caused it I believe, but they relieved his pain'.

Over a third of the mentally confused died at home. This is lower than the overall proportion in our sample, but a study in Glasgow found that only a quarter with mental abnormality died at home.[1] Most of those with mental confusion who died in a hospital or institution had been mentally confused before their admission, but 15% of the mentally confused became so only after they had gone into hospital.

A third of the mentally confused in our sample had been bedridden or confined mainly to bed for three months or more, compared with one in seven of the others who died.[2] In addition, those with mental confusion were more than twice as likely as those with other symptoms to have had bedsores (27% compared with 12%), and to have been incontinent (45% compared with 21% suffered from loss of bowel control). Fewer were said to have suffered from pain (67% against 78%); this may be because some of them communicated their feelings less effectively. It was also probably a reflection of their more advanced age and the cause of death. Half of the mentally confused were 75 or more and nearly a quarter of them died from cerebrovascular disease (stroke). (Of those without mental confusion a third were 75 or more and one in eight died from stroke.)

Most of the mentally confused, 90%, had needed help with looking after themselves while they were at home. In addition, 67% of the mentally confused had needed some attention at night compared with 43% of those with other symptoms; and the proportions needing some nursing care were 77% compared with 57%.

Relatives and friends were usually mobilised to help with these needs, and the district nurse had visited half of the patients with mental confusion. But, as other studies have also

[1] Isaacs, Bernard, *et al.*, 'The concept of pre-death'.

[2] Those who died unexpectedly before they were 65 have been excluded from this comparison.

shown, the care of mentally disturbed persons at home often caused much strain and anxiety.[1]

> 'He was getting too much for my mother-in-law to deal with. He was getting very senile and confused—insisted on going to work. Would go to work in an overcoat, then would forget to bring it home. In the winter, for instance, he'd go to work in a thin jacket and they would send him home in someone's coat to keep him warm.' (He died of pneumonia in hospital.)

It may be that relatives and friends find mental confusion more easy to come to terms with when it is associated with physical illness.

> 'It was terrible trying to cope with her at home. She seemed to be very mischievous, it took me a long time to come to terms with her. We often said, if only she'd been physically ill, we could have managed. I was a nurse and my sister was too.' . . . 'She used to hide things of importance like letters about patients I was asked to visit. One letter turned up behind a book-case two years later. She hid things so well that I couldn't believe she didn't know what she was doing.'

Often the behaviour of mentally confused people was unpredictable. They might appear perfectly clear and stable to some people who did not see them too much, but would change at times, as in the case of an 84-year-old woman whose granddaughter told us the circumstances under which she was taken into hospital.

> 'I had a few words with our doctor and he thought we could manage but then when he actually saw her bite me he changed his mind. She had to be strapped in a chair, she was really violent after the first cerebral haemorrhage so we were very relieved when she went into hospital.'

And after they were admitted there were still problems to be coped with:

> 'She complained of the staff at ——. Said they ill-treated her and took her knickers away. We kept sending new

[1] Isaacs, Bernard *et al.*, *Survival of the Unfittest*, pp. 57–61.

pairs. After she died we found at least three dozen pairs in her drawer!!'

Some of these instances may seem a bit dramatic. The illustration given by a man of his 78-year-old wife's mental confusion is less striking and perhaps more representative of the mental confusion that many people may encounter and find difficult to discuss.

> 'It started in 1963. She said she had wind so we went to Dr —— and all he could say was, "get her weight down". Well, she'd always been a big woman so that wasn't easy. She just sat about all day unless I took her out in the wheelchair. After a bit she got past going out and stayed in bed all day. She didn't talk much, but what she did say was all in the past, way back when the children were little. I asked the doctor what was wrong with her. He said, "She's a cabbage". "That's a funny thing to say", I thought, "what are you getting at?" I suppose he meant her brain was disintegrating—not registering. She had a glazy look.' (His wife died of a cerebral haemorrhage in hospital.)

When people become mentally confused before their death this may lead to a process of disengagement with their relatives. Husbands, wives, daughters and sons may take over the responsibilities of the confused people. As the relatives find they cannot rely on the confused people to perform their usual tasks their relationship will change. Relatives may withdraw to some extent and tend to feel less emotionally dependent on the person who is dying. This is in marked contrast to the situation described at the beginning of the next section.

Young deaths

Thirty-five people in our sample, 4%, died before they were 45. Six of them died unexpectedly without any previous illness or warning. Their relatives had no time for preparatory grief.[1] Five of the six were married men between 35 and 44, three men died of acute myocardial infarction and two in traffic accidents.

[1] Kubler-Ross, Elisabeth, *On Death and Dying*, p. 152. This is discussed later in Chapter 10.

'My husband was all right when he went to bed at 11.45. Then he said he had a pain in the chest. I gave him a cup of tea and an aspirin. I got hold of the doctor at ten minutes to one but he didn't come until ten minutes to two. My husband said "You could die while you're waiting for a doctor". I think he was dead when the doctor came in.'

All these five men had children under 15. Their young widows faced problems of loneliness, financial worries, anxieties about their children, ill health and difficulties about getting jobs as well as their emotional reactions to grief and bereavement.[1]

'I think the biggest problem is loneliness. If you are asked out at all you can't go regularly because of the problem of baby sitting for the children. I think it's very important to have some interest outside the home. The children are in bed by eight o'clock. The evening drags on so slowly if you just sit on your own.'

This woman had three daughters under 15 and went on to say:

'The pension relating to your husband's earnings goes on for six months. I don't think six months is long enough to get together again so to speak. They could give you more help finding the job you want to do. You can get assistance but they could help you to find work while your children are at school. They pay out too easily. I could go on drawing money indefinitely. It's four months now I've just been sitting. If someone had come round and offered to help me find work I would have been eager to do so. It's so important to give your children time as well—they've lost one parent. It is important to find a part-time job that fits in with the children's schooling.'

Another widow who also had three children under 15 made a different point about her pension:

'I just wonder why the Social Security leave me with £7 10*s*. 0*d*. widow's pension for myself and three children. When I applied for more I got supplementary for a while. But now I won't show them my bank book because in —— [husband's firm] you get 12 months' pay in a lump

[1] See Marris, Peter, *Widows and their Families*.

sum so because of that I don't get anything from the Social Security, I just get the pension plus family allowance.'

One widow was hurt in the same car crash that killed her husband. When she came home after being in hospital for six months her daughter said 'She badly needed help for nerves apart from treatment for her physical injuries. She is still terribly upset and every now and then she says she wants to move as everything reminds her of Daddy'.

One young woman who died unexpectedly committed suicide by coal gas poisoning. One man killed himself but this was not entirely unexpected as he had had two nervous breakdowns and spoken of the possibility to his wife. He had taken an overdose of sleeping pills but had not been to see his general practitioner during the last twelve months of his life. His wife explained 'I used to go and get a repeat prescription of sleeping pills and Librium. He didn't even go himself'.

Only one of the younger people who died had been in hospital for a year or more—a boy of 17 who had muscular dystrophy. He had been in an orthopaedic hospital for three years.

A rather high proportion of the young deaths in our sample were due to cancer—a half.[1] Many of them had been ill for some time and needed to be looked after during this time. About two-fifths of the young people who died of cancer had been mainly confined to bed for three months or longer compared with one-fifth of the young deaths from other causes. This could give their relatives an opportunity to prepare for their bereavement.

A woman of 41 had died of cancer after being confined mainly to bed for over a year. She had been in hospital on four different occasions during the last year but had spent more than half of it at home with her husband and three children, the youngest of whom was eleven. The district nurse had been 'coming once a day and always said how busy she was—sort of warned you off'. This was the reaction of the woman's husband who would have liked the nurse to have come more often and would also have liked

[1] This compares with an expected proportion of a quarter—see Appendix I for a discussion of this bias.

the health visitor to come again after the one visit she had made. 'She could have come in to talk to my wife. She got very depressed. She was by herself for too long a period. She would have liked company from anybody. I changed to night work so that I could be at home during the day while my sons were away. It also meant more money which helped with the housekeeping.' His wife had been 'taken into hospital the last time because she had taken an overdose'. She recovered from that but never came home again. 'About two weeks before she died we had a little conversation and she said to look after the boys and to marry again if I wanted to.'

A man who died at 42 from cancer had been completely bedridden for three to four months. His wife described how 'it was a gradual process. A lot of people would have been in bed a lot longer than he was, he had a very strong will. He used to have treatment [radiotherapy] and go to work. He was kept going by thinking the treatment would help.' His wife had looked after him at home until two months before he died when she became ill. 'I intended keeping him at home but I was taken ill so he had to go into hospital.' Her experience of support from community services was varied. 'Our doctor was ill. His partner came and said "There's no point in visiting your husband, there's nothing we can do for him". I changed to another doctor and he was marvellous. He put my husband's mind at rest. He was a help to the family too. If you've got some moral support you can carry on. He visited him once a week in hospital. He became a friend. He bothered about the children and got in touch with the headmaster and things like that.' A district nurse had come in daily for two months and the doctor arranged for a night nurse from the Marie Curie foundation to come on two occasions, but the wife could have done with a home help too. 'It was a tremendous strain, being with him night and day. Shopping and cooking was difficult. I didn't like leaving him. It would have been marvellous just to have someone to make a cup of tea.'

Earlier we showed that pain was more often reported for

people who died when they were relatively young and more often for those dying of cancer. A grandmother described the symptoms of a 17-year-old boy who died of cancer:

> 'The flesh just dropped off him. He couldn't eat at the end. The pain was terrible—he used to scream with it.' He was also depressed. 'He didn't want to see his pals in the end. They used to come and talk about what they were doing outside. He just couldn't stand it.' He had died at home, five weeks after being discharged from hospital. He lived with his mother, aunt, two sisters and three brothers, the youngest of whom was eleven. 'It was terrible to see him. It was awful for the children. It was better for him [dying at home] but it was a great ordeal for the family.'

As with the elderly, the circumstances in which young people died varied widely—although the 'case-mix' was rather different. The main distinguishing features in the impact of their illness and death were the involvement of children, their family responsibilities—social, emotional and financial—and a sense of frustration and injustice.

This somewhat diffuse and descriptive chapter has, we hope, given some idea of the variety of needs of people in the last year of their lives and the problems and conflicts posed by their care. Desires for people to spend their last days in their homes may need to be offset by needs for intensive and expert nursing and medical care and the burden their home care places on relatives. Wishes to remain independent can lead to exposure to risks of accident and neglect. The ways in which these differing needs are met or overlooked by present services are described in the following chapters.

4

HOSPITAL AND INSTITUTIONAL CARE

Just over half, 52%, of the people in our sample[1] died in a hospital or institution. Another 18% were in-patients at some time during the year before they died. The length of time people spent in hospital during the last year of their lives is shown in Table 23.

TABLE 23 *Length of time in hospital or institution during the last year*

Length of time in hospital or institution	%
Not at all	30
Less than a week	12
One week but less than a month	21
One month but less than 3 months	19
Three months but less than 6 months	7
Six months but less than a year	2
A year or more	9
Number of deaths (=100%)	781

Nine per cent of the people who died spent at least the twelve months before they did so in a hospital or institution. This included 2% who had been in for between one and two years, 4% for between two and five years, and 3% for more than five years. Only 2% were in hospital for more than six months

[1] This is based on the information collected at the interview and relates to the 785 for whom a complete interview was obtained. See Appendix IV for a comparison of data from the interview and the death certificate. A relatively high proportion of the deaths in the sample occurred in people's own homes—41% compared with 35% of all deaths in 1969. (This is discussed in the introduction and in Appendix I.)

but less than a year, so the great majority, 89%, were at home for most of the year.

In this chapter we compare the people who died in hospital with those who died at home, look at the different sorts of hospital and institution in which people died and then at the people who were in hospital at some time during the year but did not die there. After that the care of patients who will be dead within a year is viewed from the perspective of the hospitals and institutions. An estimate is made of the proportion of bed-days taken up by 'dying' patients.

Who dies in hospital?

In the introduction we showed, from national statistics, that people dying of cancer, stroke, respiratory disease and particularly those dying from relatively uncommon causes were more likely to die in hospital than those with other types of circulatory disease or accidents. There was little difference in the proportions of men and women dying in N.H.S. hospitals or other institutions for the care of the sick, but rather more women than men died in private or other institutions, 8·4% against 3·9%. Table 24 shows where the people in our sample

TABLE 24 *Place of death by age at death*

	Age at death					
Place of death (interview data)	15–44	45–54	55–64	65–74	75–84	85+
	%	%	%	%	%	%
Hospital	66	40	46	46	46	46
Other institution	—	—	3	5	5	12
Person's own home[a]	31	53	43	41	44	36
Other person's home	—	2	3	3	3	4
Other	3	5	5	5	2	2
Number of deaths (=100%)	35	55	145	238	213	98

[a] This was their usual home, and if they lived permanently with, for example, a married daughter and her family, this was counted as their home.

died and their ages. (Such an analysis is not published by the Office of Population Censuses and Surveys.)

Those dying when they were under 45 were the ones most likely to die in hospital. The proportion dying in other institutions increased with age. Over half those aged 45–54 died in their own home, and this proportion fell to just over a third of those aged 85 or more.

Household composition was clearly related to the place of death (see Table 25). The proportion dying in hospital was highest, three-fifths, for those who lived alone, but still a quarter of those who lived alone died in their own homes. Hospital deaths and deaths in their own homes were equally divided among those living just with their wife or husband while among those living with children or other relatives of a younger generation home deaths were slightly more common than deaths in hospital. Those living with unmarried daughters were more likely to die in their own home than those living with unmarried sons: 60% compared with 34%. (This difference persisted whether or not they also lived with their spouse.) But there was no difference in the proportion dying at home between those living with married daughters and those

TABLE 25 *Place of death and household composition*

	Household composition				
Place of death (interview data)	*On own*	*With spouse (with or without relatives of same or older generation)*	*With relatives of same or older generation only*	*With relatives of younger generation (with or without spouse)*	*With unrelated people*
	%	%	%	%	%
Hospital	59	46	54	41	46
Other institution	9	1	9	2	31[a]
Person's own home	25	47	32	49	17
Other person's home	3	2	5	4	—
Other	4	4	—	4	6
Number of deaths (=100%)	118	244	44	329	48

[a] Includes a number of people living in guesthouses who died there.

TABLE 26 *Place of death, sex and marital status*

Place of death (interview data)	Men				Women			
	Single	*Married*	*Widowed etc.*	*All men*	*Single*	*Married*	*Widowed etc.*	*All women*
	%	%	%	%	%	%	%	%
Hospital	49	42	50	45	44	49	47	48
Other institution	12	1	7	4	21	2	6	6
Person's own home	32	50	36	44	27	45	38	39
Other person's home	2	2	3	2	6	2	6	4
Elsewhere	5	5	4	5	2	2	3	3
Number of deaths (=100%)	41	271	100	418[a]	52	129	179	367[a]

[a] Includes the few whose marital status was not known.

TABLE 27 *Place of death and living children*

Place of death (interview data)	*Children*						
	One son only	*One daughter only*	*Sons only*	*Daughters only*	*Son(s) and daughter(s)*	*Any children*	*No children*
	%	%	%	%	%	%	%
Hospital	55	42	63	37	41	45	47
Other institution	2	1	2	2	—	1	6
Person's own home	40	54	28	59	52	48	39
Other person's home	3	3	5	2	3	3	5
Elsewhere	—	—	2	—	4	3	3
Number of deaths (=100%)[a]	63	90	60	49	230	492	144

[a] Excluding those who had been in hospital or other institution for a year or more before they died and those who died unexpectedly, as information was not collected about the children of these people.

with married sons. Deaths in other institutions occurred mainly among those living on their own, with people not related to them, or with relatives (but not their spouse) of the same generation.

Associated with these differences were the variations with sex and marital status shown in Table 26.

Single people and particularly single women were relatively likely to die in an institution, while married people and particularly married men were most likely to die in their own homes. However, further analyses suggested that the reason for the variation in place of death was the existence of children rather than marital status. When those with no children were compared there was no difference in the place of death between those who were single, married or widowed.[1] Those with children more often died in their own homes than those with no children: 48% compared with 39% (see Table 27).

People who had a daughter or daughters were more likely to die at home than those who had just a son or sons. This can be seen from Table 27. There was some suggestion that more of those with just one son died at home than those with two or more sons but no daughters, but this difference might have occurred by chance. Another study[2] suggested 'stronger ties of mutual affection or a stronger sense of obligation on the part of only children'.

It is perhaps surprising that those dying in hospital should differ so little in their number of symptoms from those dying in their own homes (see Table 28). The average number varied little except for those dying in 'other places' such as the street, their office, or when they were away on holiday. This group contained a relatively high proportion of unexpected deaths.

The nature of their symptoms was slightly different. Those who died in hospital were more likely to suffer from pain and mental confusion, while vomiting, loss of appetite, trouble with breathing and bedsores were more common among those who died at home. It is likely that relatives were more aware of these symptoms when people were at home. Incontinence was no

[1] Information about children was not obtained for those who had been in a hospital or institution for a year or more or for those who died unexpectedly, so these have to be excluded from the comparison.

[2] Tunstall, Jeremy, *Old and Alone*, p. 51.

TABLE 28 *Symptoms and place of death*

	Place of death (interview data)				
	Hospital	*Other institution*	*Own home*	*Other person's home*	*Other*
	%	%	%	%	%
Pain	72	46	65	48	47
Sleeplessness	48	49	53	52	17
Loss of bladder control	34	41	28	61	3
Loss of bowel control	29	41	26	43	—
Unpleasant smell	16	19	15	22	—
Vomiting	28	27	35	30	3
Loss of appetite	45	41	56	35	13
Constipation	27	19	33	30	13
Bedsores	14	19	20	17	—
Mental confusion	41	49	31	52	—
Trouble with breathing	42	41	52	43	23
Depression	39	27	33	52	17
Other	28	16	23	30	13
None[a]	7	13	11	9	47
Number of deaths (=100%)	362	37	325	23	30
Average number of symptoms	4·4	3·9	4·5	4·8	1·5

[a] The questions about symptoms were not asked for the unexpected deaths of people under 65 with no reported restrictions. They have been included as having no symptoms.

more frequent among those dying in hospital than among those dying at home, but those dying in hospital had been incontinent for longer. Among the incontinent 32% of those dying in hospital had been incontinent for a year or longer, 18% of those dying at home. About a quarter of those dying in hospital who were incontinent were said to have become so after they were admitted. Isaacs and his colleagues report similar findings: they found no difference in the prevalence of incontinence among those who died at home or in hospital, but more of those dying in hospital were said to have mental abnormality.[1]

[1] Isaacs, Bernard, *et al.*, 'The concept of pre-death'.

Those dying in their own homes were slightly less disabled or restricted than those dying in hospital. The proportions with no restrictions were 18% among those dying at home and 12% among those dying in hospital. Isaacs found no difference between these two groups in the proportion with immobility.[1]

So far the main differences that have emerged between those dying at home and those dying in a hospital are in their household composition and whether or not they had any children, particularly daughters, rather than the number, severity or length of time for which they had symptoms. Pain and mental confusion were more common amongst those dying in hospital, incontinence was not. How did they differ in the extent to which they needed help while they were at home? Those who died at home were more likely to have needed help with self care, nursing and night care while they were at home than were those who died in hospital. These differences are shown in Table 29.

One problem in interpreting the data in Table 29 is that different points in time are being compared. For the people who died at home it is the help they needed just before they died, for those who died in hospital the help they needed just before they went into hospital. The table also shows that those who died in a hospital or institution had needed help with self care and night care at home for somewhat longer than those dying at home. The longer needs persist, the more chance there is of some crisis in the lives of those caring for people at home which may precipitate admission to a hospital or institution. Certainly most of those dying in a hospital or institution had needed care at home before they were admitted.

The types of hospital and institution in which people die

The types of hospital and institution recorded on the death certificates are shown in Table 30.[2]

[1] Isaacs, Bernard, *et al.*, 'The concept of pre-death'.

[2] The classification into mental hospitals or psychiatric institutions, other hospitals and institutions under the N.H.S., private hospitals and institutions for the care of the sick, and permanent places of residence of an institutional nature was done by the Office of Population Censuses and Surveys. We classified hospitals further, by using the *Hospitals Year Book 1969*, into teaching hospitals and the groups shown in the lower part of Table 30. For a description of how

TABLE 29 *Help needed and place of death*

	Place of death (interview data)		
	Hospital or institution	*Own or other person's home*	*Elsewhere*
Needed help at home with:	%	%	%
Self care	67	76	10
Nursing care	53	67	13
Night care	40	56	7
Social care	60	66	13
Financial care	21	22	20
Housework	52	46	20
None of these[a]	15	16	67
Number (=100%)[b]	328	346	30
Length of time needed help with self care at home	%	%	Numbers too small
Less than a week	12	11	
One week but less than 1 year	39	50	
One year or more	49	39	
Number needing help with self care (=100%)	205	243	
Length of time needed night care at home	%	%	
Less than a week	22	34	
One week but less than 1 year	65	53	
One year or more	13	13	
Number needing night care (=100%)	111	157	

[a] Those who died unexpectedly before they were 65 have been included as not needing help.
[b] Excluding those who had been in a hospital or institution for a year or more before they died.

Four per cent of the hospital and institutional deaths occurred in teaching hospitals—although in 1967, the latest year for

the place of death on the death certificate was related to that recorded at the interview, see Appendix IV.

which such statistics are available, 14% of all hospitals discharges and deaths were from teaching hospitals.[1] It seems that people with terminal illnesses are less likely than others to be in a teaching hospital and therefore medical students are likely

TABLE 30 *Types of institution in which people died*

	All deaths	*All institutional deaths*
Place of death (from death certificate)	%	%
Teaching hospital	2	4
Mental hospital or psychiatric institution[a]	3	6
Other N.H.S. hospital or institution	41	77
Private hospitals and nursing homes	4	7
Permanent place of residence	3	6
Own home	41	—
Elsewhere	6	—
Type of institution	%	%
Acute	22	43
Mainly or partly acute	9	18
Chronic, long-stay, geriatric	7	12
Mental illness or subnormality	3	6
Chest, T.B.	1	2
Cancer and radiotherapy Dying, terminal and advanced cases }	1	1
Other hospital (including combinations of above)	3	5
Private nursing home	4	7
Permanent institution	3	6
Not in institution	47	—
Number of deaths (=100%)	785	414

[a] Includes both N.H.S. and private hospitals and institutions.

to come into contact with death relatively rarely. People who died in teaching hospitals were more often under 65 than those who died in other general hospitals: 52% compared with 30%. Only 5% of those dying in teaching hospitals died of stroke, 19% of those in other general hospitals.

[1] Department of Health and Social Security and Office of Population Censuses and Surveys, *Report on Hospital In-patient Enquiry for the year 1967*, p. 2.

Two-fifths of the institutional deaths took place in acute hospitals and only 2% of the patients who died in such hospitals had been there or in any institution for six months or more. This proportion was similar, 3%, for those dying in partly acute hospitals. But the proportions who had been in a hospital or institution for six months or longer was 32% of those dying in private hospitals or nursing homes, 39% of those in geriatric, long-stay or chronic hospitals, 64% of those in mental illness hospitals or institutions and 82% of those in permanent institutions. And slightly over a third of those who died in a mental illness or permanent institution had been there or in some other institution for at least five years.[1]

Just over a quarter of those dying in geriatric or chronic hospitals were said to have had bedsores, less than half this proportion in the other types of hospital. Incontinence was relatively infrequent among those dying in acute or partly acute hospitals.[1]

Two-thirds of those dying in permanent institutions were 80 or more, half of those in chronic or long-stay hospitals, just over a third of those in private nursing homes and mental illness hospitals, less than a fifth of those in acute, partly acute and 'other hospitals'.

There were also large differences in marital status (see Table 31).

Half the people who died in permanent institutions, and a third of those in mental illness hospitals, had never married. As we showed earlier, a number of those dying in such places had been there for at least five years. Some may have been there nearly all their adult lives because of mental subnormality or chronic disability. Less than a fifth of those dying in all other hospitals or in private nursing homes were single, while a low proportion of those dying in mental illness hospitals or permanent institutions were married. There were also relatively few married people, about a third, in the geriatric, chronic or long-stay hospitals and private nursing homes compared with over half in acute and partly acute and 'other hospitals'. The proportion of female compared with male deaths was high, three-quarters, in private nursing homes. This is in line with

[1] Details are in Appendix IX.

TABLE 31 *Type of institution and marital status*

	Type of Institution						
	Acute	*Partly acute*	*Mental illness*	*Geriatric, long-stay, chronic*	*Other N.H.S. hospitals*	*Private hospitals or nursing homes*	*Permanent institutions*
	%	%	%	%	%	%	%
Single	13	6	33	10	15	17	50
Married	54	60	17	35	64	33	4
Widowed	31	31	50	53	21	50	46
Divorced or separated	2	3	—	2	—	—	—
Number of deaths in hospitals and institutions (=100%)	171	71	24	51	33	30	24

national statistics (see Chapter 1). There were no other significant differences.

Discharged to die

A sizeable proportion, 37%, of those who died at home had been in a hospital or institution at some time during the year before they died. Expressing this as a proportion of all the people who died, 18% had been in a hospital or institution as an in-patient at some time in the twelve months before they died but did not die there (17% died in their homes, 1% somewhere else). Many of them were apparently discharged to die. The proportion of 'expected' deaths[1] in this group was 71% compared with 59% among those dying in a hospital or institution and 39% among those dying at home or elsewhere who had not been in hospital during the previous year. A third of them had been discharged between six months and a year before they died, a quarter between three and six months, another quarter between one and three months, and a fifth within the last month of their lives.

Half the people who came home to die died of cancer. This

[1] Question 3: 'As far as you were concerned was ——'s death expected or not?'

compares with just over a quarter of those dying in hospitals or institutions and one in seven of the others. Looking at this in another way, half of those dying of cancer did so in a hospital or institution, a third died after discharge, and one in six had not been in hospital as an in-patient at all in the year before they died. Associated with this, those dying at home after discharge from hospital were comparatively young—43% were under 65 compared with 29% of those dying in hospital or institutions—and more symptoms were reported for them, particularly sleeplessness, vomiting, loss of appetite, constipation, bedsores and trouble with breathing (see Table 32). But, again, the people we interviewed were likely to be more aware of symptoms when the person was at home than when he was in hospital. However, other data also suggest that those who were discharged and died at home had many problems and needed a lot of looking after. Many of them had symptoms which were described as very disturbing—84% compared with 69% of those dying in hospital and 56% of those who had not been in hospital in the last year of their lives. The proportions needing help with all types of care (except financial) while they were at home were also greater among those discharged from hospital.

More of those discharged were married, fewer lived alone and more of them lived with relatives of a younger generation (see Table 33). So they were more likely to have families and friends able to look after them. Two-thirds of the respondents we interviewed about people who had died at home after being in hospital said they were glad the person had died at home rather than in hospital.[1] But this proportion was higher, four-fifths, when the person had died at home without ever going into hospital in the last year.

The hospitals retained some contact and responsibility for some of these discharged patients: half of them had attended hospital as out-patients more than once in the year before they died, a fifth had been on five or more occasions. And the amount of care they had from general practitioners and district nurses was greater than it was for those who died in hospital or for

[1] Question 74: 'How did you feel about —— dying at home rather than in hospital?' This question was omitted for unexpected home deaths, as well as for those not dying at home.

TABLE 32 *Circumstances of death and age, symptoms and care needed*

	Circumstances of death		
	In hospital or institution	*After discharge*	*Never in hospital*[a]
Age:	%	%	%
Under 45	6 } 29	5 } 43	2 } 24
45–54	5	13	6
55–64	18	25	16
65–74	30	33	30
75+	41	24	46
Symptoms:	%	%	%
Pain	70	77	54
Sleeplessness	48	69	38
Loss of bladder control	35	32	26
Loss of bowel control	30	32	21
Unpleasant smell	16	23	9
Vomiting	28	49	22
Loss of appetite	44	74	37
Constipation	26	40	26
Bedsores	15	25	14
Mental confusion	41	38	26
Trouble with breathing	41	56	45
Depression	38	47	26
Other	27	35	15
None[b]	8	4	19
Needed help at home with:	%[c]	%	%
Self care	67	83	64
Nursing care	54	76	55
Night care	40	65	45
Social care	61	74	54
Financial care	21	22	21
Housework	56	63	44
None of these[b]	14	9	27
Number of deaths (=100%)[d]	404	141	236

[a] During the twelve months before they died.

[b] Those who died unexpectedly when they were under 65 with no previous restrictions are included as having no symptoms and needing no help.

[c] Excluding those who had been in hospitals or institutions all the year—so the base for these percentages was 332.

[d] Those for whom inadequate information was obtained have been excluded when calculating percentages.

TABLE 33 *Circumstances of death and marital status, sex, household composition and general practitioner and district nursing care*

	Circumstances of death		
	In hospital or institution	*After discharge*	*Never in hospital*[a]
Marital status at time of death:	%	%	%
Married	46	64	54
Single	15	10	9
Widowed, etc.	39	26	37
Sex:	%	%	%
Male	50	61	53
Female	50	39	47
Household composition:	%	%	%
On own	20	5	13
With spouse only	27	32	32
With relatives of same or older generation only[b]	9	6	6
With relatives of a younger generation[b]	35	55	45
With unrelated people or in guest-house	9	2	4
General practitioner consultations in last twelve months:	%[c]	%	%
Not at all	3	0	9
1–4	25	11	24
5–9	24	14	18
10–19	25	27	24
20+	23	48	25
Proportion who had been visited by a district nurse at home	24%[c]	53%	35%
Number of deaths (=100%)[d]	404	141	236

[a] During the twelve months before they died.
[b] With or without spouse.
[c] Excluding those who had been in hospitals or institutions all the year—so the base for these percentages was 332.
[d] Those for whom inadequate information was obtained have been excluded when calculating percentages.

those dying at home who had not been in hospital during the year before they died.

For these patients the dilemmas of caring for people with terminal illness were particularly intense. They had many problems and needed a great deal of care, often over a long period. Others with similar needs but no relatives or friends who could look after them could not be discharged home and had to be cared for in hospitals or institutions. The burden on relatives who took responsibility for the care of people discharged to die was heavy, and a third of these relatives were either uncertain that it was appropriate for the person to have died at home or thought it would have been better for him to have been in hospital.

Implications

Data from the Hospital In-patients Enquiry which covers National Health Service hospitals in England and Wales[1] show that in 1969 deaths accounted for 5·5% of the discharges and deaths. People who died in hospital had spent an average of sixty days in hospital during the spell that preceded their death, compared with an average stay of 12·5 days for other patients.[2] It is not possible to calculate precisely from these data what proportion of hospital bed-days were taken up by patients who died there, because the average length of stay is likely to be inflated by a small proportion of patients with long stays, some of which will exceed a year. If this problem is ignored, calculations indicate that 22% of the bed-days were taken up by people who died there. (Data from the present survey cannot be used to estimate the lengths of stay in particular types of hospital because only the type of hospital in which people died was classified and the length of stay related to the time spent in any hospital or institution before they died. The estimated average length of stay for those dying in N.H.S. hospitals apart from mental illness ones was sixty-one days—counting those in hospital for a year or more as having a length of stay of 365 days.)

[1] Excluding hospitals confined to the treatment of subnormality and other psychiatric diseases.

[2] Office of Population Censuses and Surveys. Unpublished reference table giving type of case and mean duration of stay.

A number of people dying in hospital would have been in hospital on other occasions during the year before their death. We found that 33% of people in our sample who died in hospital had been in hospital for more than one spell during the last twelve months of their lives. They averaged 1·4 other spells. In addition 37% of the people who died at home had been in hospital at some stage during the year before their death.

If we make the following rather crude assumptions, it is possible to make a rough estimate of the proportion of hospital bed-days 'consumed' by people who would be dead within a year. The assumptions are:

1. All the people who died at home but who had been in hospital for some time during the twelve months before their death were in N.H.S. hospitals—other than mental illness ones. (This seems reasonable in view of their ages, causes of death, etc.)
2. The average length of time these people spent in hospital was forty-two days. (This is estimated from our interview data.)
3. The average additional time spent in hospital during the year by people who died there was 17·5 days. (This is probably an under-estimate as it is based on an average length of stay of 12·5 days.)

On these assumptions we find that 2% of hospital bed-days are taken up by people who do not die there during that spell but die in hospital during another admission within twelve months. And 5% of bed-days are taken up by people who die at home within the year. Taken together with the estimate of 22% of bed-days taken up by people dying in hospital, these figures suggest that between a quarter and three-tenths of hospital bed-days in a year are taken up by people who will be dead within twelve months.[1] This represents a large amount of resources. As hospitals account for nearly three-fifths of the

[1] In 1950–3 a study of male patients discharged from medical units of four 'acute' hospitals in the west of Scotland found that two years later a quarter of them were dead. See Ferguson, Thomas and MacPhail, A. N., *Hospital and Community*, p. 81.

expenditure on health and welfare services, it means that something like 15% of all this expenditure is devoted to the hospital care of people who will be dead within twelve months. That is appreciably more than the *total* amount spent on local authority health services.[1]

This study and others raise a number of doubts about the appropriateness of the care that these people receive.

As the care of people who will soon be dead forms such a large part of hospital work, the amount of specialisation in this type of care seems small. There are a few hospitals and institutions which specialise in terminal care[2] (less than 1% of the people in our sample died in such places). It is important that the expertise developed in such places for the relief of pain and other distressing symptoms and in creating a pleasant atmosphere for dying patients and their relatives should be recognised and more widely disseminated in geriatric departments, acute wards and in general practice. Medical schools and teaching hospitals should devote more of their resources to the development of these skills.

But are acute hospitals the most suitable places in which to care for many of these patients? It may be that many such patients are sent there because no other, more appropriate, sources of care are available. In 1949 Lowe and McKeown found that many patients were retained in hospital 'whose need for frequent medical attention or skilled nursing was transient, but whose home circumstances prevented discharge'.[3] More recent studies suggest that this is still so twenty years later.[4]

It is clear from the present study that social needs affect both hospital admission and discharge. This suggests that homes providing nursing care could meet the needs of many of the patients at present cared for in hospitals with all their technical facilities. At the moment the hospital services appear to be caring for people who in different social conditions would be

[1] Department of Health and Social Security, *Annual Report 1970.*

[2] Saunders, Cicely M. S., 'The treatment of intractable pain in terminal cancer' and 'The care of the terminal stages of cancer'.

[3] Lowe, C. R. and McKeown, Thomas, 'The care of the chronic sick: medical and nursing requirements'.

[4] Butler, John R. and Pearson, Mary, *Who Goes Home?*

looked after at home by relatives with the support of some community services. Are the decisions made on this basis informed and appropriate? Some light is thrown on this by the experience and views of general practitioners through whom most hospital admissions are arranged.

5

THE GENERAL PRACTITIONER

This chapter starts by describing the amount and intensity of care given by general practitioners to people in the last year of their lives. It goes on to show that in spite of frequent contact with most people in the year before they died the general practitioner was often not consulted about such symptoms as an unpleasant smell, loss of bladder control and depression. Analysis of the experiences of patients and their relationships with their doctors reveal some reasons for this.

The general practitioner's role as an instigator of hospital care and co-ordinator of community services is then examined. Most general practitioners felt that N.H.S. facilities for old people in need of long-term nursing care were inadequate. They were more complacent, although sometimes ignorant, about community services.

Care in the last year

People who did not spend all the last year of their lives in a hospital or institution tended to have several contacts with their general practitioners during that time. Table 34 shows that over half of them were said to have had ten or more consultations.[1] The figures are based on information from relatives and friends. It will have been difficult for them to recall the facts accurately and they may not have been aware of all the consultations that took place.

Many of the consultations were home visits. Over a quarter of the people who died had had at least one night call, one in

[1] This compares with under a quarter of people aged 75 or more on a general survey found to have so many consultations. See Cartwright, Ann, *Patients and their Doctors*, p. 187. And a study by Townsend of people 'of pensionable age' found that a quarter of the men and a sixth of the women had consulted their doctor more than ten times in a year. Townsend, Peter, *The Family Life of Old People*, p. 51.

TABLE 34 *General practitioner consultations*

All consultations	%
0	4
1–4	22
5–9	20
10–19	25
20+	29
Home visits	%
0	12
1–4	31
5–9	17
10–19	17
20+	23
Night calls—between 8 p.m. and 8 a.m.	%
0	73
1	17
2–4	7
5+	3
Number of deaths excluding those who had been in hospital or institution for a year or more (=100%)[a]	713

[a] Those for whom inadequate information was obtained are included in the total but have been excluded when calculating percentages.

ten more than one. Even so, 52% of the people who *died at home* had no night calls and 30% less than five home visits.

A comparatively high proportion of those dying of cancer had ten or more consultations: 70% compared with 44% of those dying from other causes. But they did not have significantly more home visits or night calls.

There was no clear trend with age in the total number of general practitioner consultations, but the proportion who had ten or more *home visits* from a general practitioner in a year rose from 33% of those under 65 to 61% of those who were 85 or more. Three-fifths of the women had ten or more consultations during the year, rather less, half, of the men had so many. People who lived alone appeared to have less contact with their general practitioner than others. Sixteen per cent of them were said to have consulted their doctor twenty or more times in the last year of their lives, in contrast to 30% of people living with others. Eighteen per cent of those living alone received no home visits compared with 11% of others, and only 11% had any night visits against 29% of people not living alone. Part of the explanation for this last difference may be the difficulty of getting in touch with the doctor when you are ill and live alone. A fifth of the people who lived alone had a telephone compared with nearly two-fifths of those living with others, and people with telephones were more likely to have had a visit at night than those without—33% against 26%. Another reason for people living alone having fewer contacts with general practitioners was that, as we saw earlier in Chapter 2, they were reported to have fewer restrictions than others,[1] and they were also more likely to be admitted to a hospital or institution. But the consultations of people living alone may have been under-reported, as the person interviewed did not live in the same household and may not have known about some of the consultations.

The extent of morbidity, as indicated by reported symptoms, that general practitioners were caring for is illustrated by comparing patients who had less than five consultations with those who had five to nineteen, and those having twenty or more. This is done in Table 35.

The reported morbidity among those with twenty or more consultations was appreciably higher than among those who died in hospital. (Some patients were in both groups.) Data in the previous chapter suggest that this was related to the discharge of patients with high morbidity. General practitioners' views on the arrangements for admission and discharge of patients are discussed later in this chapter. Before that we consider the extent to which doctors were consulted about different symptoms.

Relief of symptoms

People developed most of their symptoms at home. (About one in seven of those with mental confusion, one in six of those

[1] Unfortunately our numbers are too small to do a useful analysis of consultation rates with household composition, extent of restriction and age.

TABLE 35 *Symptoms, help needed and general practitioner consultations*

	Number of general practitioner consultations in last 12 months of life		
	0–4	*5–19*	*20+*
Symptoms	%	%	%
Pain	53	74	75
Sleeplessness	25	53	73
Loss of bladder control	15	33	40
Loss of bowel control	13	29	37
Unpleasant smell	8	14	22
Vomiting	18	31	48
Loss of appetite	25	55	68
Constipation	15	31	44
Bedsores	6	17	28
Mental confusion	23	32	47
Trouble with breathing	31	50	60
Depression	21	40	46
Other	18	26	32
None[a]	29	4	2
Average number of symptoms	2·6	4·6	5·9
Restrictions	%	%	%
Bedridden for a year or more	—	2	6
Bedridden or confined to bed 3 months or more	10	15	30
Severely restricted 3 months or more	10	18	17
Moderately restricted 3 months or more	13	17	16
Other restrictions 3 months or more	11	18	13
Bedridden or confined to bed less than 3 months	15	18	10
Other restrictions less than 3 months	2	2	3
None	39	10	5
Number of deaths excluding those in hospital or institution for a year or more before they died (=100%)[b]	170	294	187

[a] Those who died unexpectedly before they were 65 with no previous restrictions have been included here.

[b] Those for whom inadequate information was obtained have been excluded when calculating percentages.

with double incontinence and a quarter of those with bedsores developed them after they were admitted to a hospital or institution, but only 5% of all other symptoms developed after admission.) When the person suffered from the symptom at

TABLE 36 *Care of symptoms*

	Pain	*Sleeplessness*	*Loss of bladder control only*	*Loss of bowel control only*	*Loss of bowel and bladder control*	*Unpleasant smell*	*Vomiting*	*Loss of appetite*	*Constipation*	*Bedsores*	*Mental confusion*	*Breathing trouble*	*Depression*	*Other*
Proportion of total sample who had symptom														
(a) in hospital or institution only	2%	1%	1%	—	4%	1%	2%	2%	1%	4%	5%	3%	2%	2%
(b) at home	64%	48%	7%	4%	20%	14%	28%	46%	27%	12%	31%	42%	34%	23%
Number of people (=100%)	← 785[a] →													
Proportion with symptom at home who consulted:	%	%	%	%	%	%	%	%	%	%	%	%	%	%
General practitioner	88	80	43	49	57	33	76	51	61	54	62	82	52	70
Hospital doctor	11	4	7	4	7	4	9	4	5	1	4	7	7	9
Hospital sister or nurse	—	—	—	—	1	—	—	1	1	—	—	—	—	1
District nurse	—	—	4	11	17	7	1	1	5	42	1	—	—	1
Other person	—	—	4	8	1	—	—	—	1	—	—	—	—	1
No one	7	17	54	29	25	58	21	45	30	17	35	14	42	22
Number with symptom at home (=100%)[b]	476	338	54	28	135	92	201	308	192	90	218	283	212	167

[a] Those for whom inadequate information was obtained have been excluded when calculating percentages.
[b] Some of the percentages add to more than 100 as more than one person was sometimes consulted about a symptom.

home we asked if he had sought any advice about it and if so from whom.[1] Replies are shown in Table 36. The general practitioner was by far the most frequent source of advice. He had been consulted about nearly two-thirds of all reported symptoms. But no help had been sought for a quarter of the symptoms and this proportion was over half for an unpleasant smell and loss of bladder but not bowel control. It was two-fifths for depression and over a quarter for loss of bowel control. We do not know how often the doctor remained unaware of these symptoms when people did not ask him about them directly.

One reason for not consulting the doctor might have been that symptoms were felt to be relatively trivial or of short duration. Certainly this seemed to be part of the explanation—but not the complete one. Twenty-nine per cent of all the symptoms about which no advice had been sought were described as 'very distressing' and 37% had been present for a year or more. Comparable proportions for symptoms for which general practitioner advice had been sought were 53% regarded as 'very distressing' and 50% present for a year or more.

When people had sought advice about the various symptoms did they feel the general practitioner or other people they asked had been able to help? The proportion who thought the person had obtained some help or relief as a result of advice[2] varied from 21% of those consulting about an unpleasant smell, 43% about loss of appetite and 44% about mental confusion to 87% about pain, 86% about sleeplessness and 81% about constipation. Obviously one of the main reasons for people not consulting was a realistic assessment of the probable outcome. The relationship between the proportion consulting and the proportion of those consulting who had been helped is shown in Figure 1 for the thirteen symptoms. The correlation coefficient is 0·80 ($p. < 0{\cdot}01$). This was reflected in some of their comments when asked why they had not sought advice.[3]

> 'Knew he couldn't do anything.' (Loss of appetite—had sarcoma of femur.)

[1] Question 42d: 'Did he or you ask anyone's advice about it? Whom did you or he ask?'

[2] Question 42c(ii): 'Were they able to help in any way?'

[3] Question 42f: 'Why didn't you or he ask for advice?'

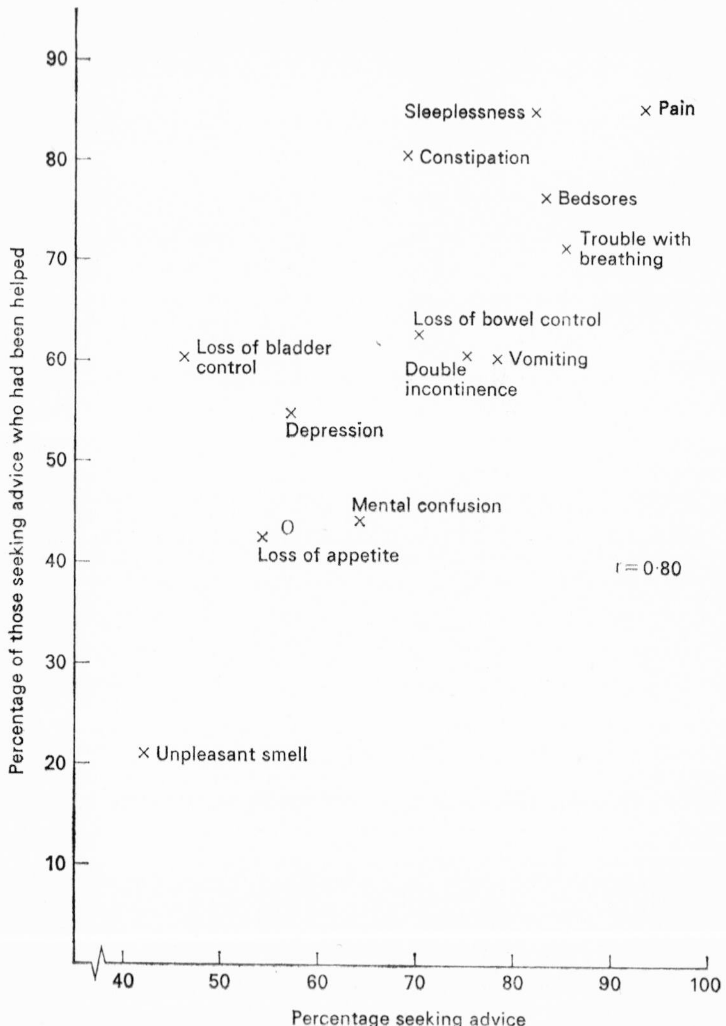

FIGURE I *Relationship between proportion consulting about different symptoms and proportion helped when they did consult*

'It was part of his illness and nothing could be done for his condition.' (Depression—had cancer of prostate.)

Many things were 'accepted as part of the condition'. For instance, the daughter of a man with Parkinson's disease said about his depression: 'We thought it was natural. We knew it was all to do with his condition.' But about the unpleasant smell: 'We never discussed it. Mother was distressed.' Embarrassment may have been the reason for some people not raising the question of incontinence with a doctor.

Some of the people who died did not seem to want to discuss their problems with a doctor and had involved their relatives and friends in a conspiracy of silence.

One woman with a breast cancer and seven different symptoms had not consulted the doctor about any of them. Her housekeeper said 'I was threatened by her not to tell a soul about her breast—not even her husband. I kept it to myself. She refused to see a doctor. We pleaded with her. It did worry me. I know now she thought he would find out about her breast.'

A woman whose husband had pain, sleeplessness, vomiting, trouble with breathing and depression and had not consulted the doctor about any of them said: 'I don't really know why. I think he really didn't want to know. I was afraid to cause trouble. I was afraid of upsetting my husband if I fussed too much. I only spoke to his sisters—he was funny about the doctor. The doctor said I should have gone to him myself and he would have come to see him. His brothers and sister begged him to go to the doctor but he wouldn't'. (Died of coronary thrombosis.)

When the doctor gave the impression that he was busy or uninterested it seemed that people were rather less likely to seek his advice. A general practitioner was consulted about 61% of the symptoms when relatives said the doctor did not have time to discuss things, compared with 70% of the symptoms when they felt he had time, or gave a qualified answer to this question.[1]

[1] Question 24: 'Do you think he has time to discuss things or not?'

The general practitioner and the hospital

In a study about ten years earlier Hughes concluded that 'there should be a much greater readiness on the part of medical and lay staff to admit to acute beds those patients entering into the final stage of their illness, who can be regarded as acute in their need for a high standard of nursing care and the ready availability of medical staff to supervise their medical needs, especially the relief of pain.'[1] Rather more recently, in 1965–6, Warren, *et al.* found that older people experience difficulty in obtaining emergency admissions.[2] What was the position at the time of the present survey? We asked the general practitioners whether they usually found it easy, rather difficult or very difficult to arrange admission into a suitable N.H.S. institution for the various sorts of people listed in Table 37.

The general practitioners experienced most difficulty in placing an old person needing long-term nursing care. And whereas 71% of the doctors said they found it easy to arrange admission for a *young* patient with a terminal illness likely to be

TABLE 37 *General practitioners' experience of the difficulty of getting admission into a suitable N.H.S. institution for various groups of patients*

	A young patient with a short-term terminal illness	*An old patient with a short-term terminal illness*	*An old person likely to need long-term nursing care*	*A young person with a progressive degenerative condition*	*An old patient with an acute infection*
Usually:	%	%	%	%	%
Easy	71	28	10	29	58
Rather difficult	22	46	37	47	31
Very difficult	6	24	51	23	7
Qualified	1	2	2	1	4
Number of doctors (=100%)[a]			323		

[a] A few who gave inadequate replies were omitted when the percentages were calculated.

[1] Hughes, H. L. Glyn, *Peace at the Last.*

[2] Warren, M. D., Cooper, J. and Warren, J. L., 'Problems of emergency admissions to London hospitals'.

of short duration, this proportion was 28% when they were seeking admission for an old patient with a similar problem.

The majority of doctors, 85%, thought there was adequate consultation between them and hospital medical staff about the admission of patients. Fifteen per cent were critical.

> 'I personally use the Emergency Bed Service. I've long since given up getting through to the hospital direct. You make phone call after phone call. It's time wasting and you more often than not get a refusal from some junior doctor in the end. I leave it to the E.B.S. to sort it out.'

Those who felt there was inadequate consultation between general practitioners and hospital medical staff about admission were more likely to report difficulties in getting patients admitted: their average score on estimated difficulty of securing admission[1] was 4·8, compared with 3·9 who felt consultation was adequate.

Most general practitioners saw their difficulties in obtaining admission for their patients as the result of inadequate numbers of beds rather than inadequate consultation with hospital staff. When asked whether they thought more of a number of facilities[2] were needed in their area, geriatric beds and chronic hospital beds were most often mentioned (see Table 38).

Some comments were:

> 'Geriatric beds are extremely difficult to come by—especially long-term beds.'

> 'Geriatric beds—especially for short-term, e.g. holiday periods for relatives. It's impossible for them to get away even with increased home help.'

> 'Geriatric assessment beds: I don't want to keep them in there, just for assessment.'

[1] Those who said it was very difficult to secure admission scored '2' each time they said this, those who said it was rather difficult '1' and those who said it was easy '0'. The score therefore ranged from 0 to 10. The average was 4·0.

[2] G.P. Question 3: 'In your area which if any of these do you think you need more of: short-term general hospital beds, chronic hospital beds, geriatric beds, mental hospital places, district nurse services, home help services, none?' Question 4: 'Which *one* do you feel is needed most?'

TABLE 38 *General practitioners' views on facilities needed in their area*

	Needed at all	*Needed most*
	%	%
Short-term general hospital beds	47	8
Chronic hospital beds	86	29
Geriatric beds	89	51
Mental hospital places	34	2
District nurse services	24	2
Home help services	55	8
Number of general practitioners (=100%)	319	303

One of the ways in which general practitioners sometimes facilitate hospital admission for their patients is by arranging for a specialist consultant to pay a domiciliary visit.[1] Table 39 shows that the number of domiciliary consultations was greater when they had more difficulty in arranging admission.[2]

Similar proportions of patients dying at home and in hospital had a domiciliary consultation. Altogether 14% of the patients had such a visit in the twelve months before they died.[3] Whether or not they had one did not seem to be related to their age, household composition or cause of death, but it rose from 6% of those in Social Class V, the unskilled workers, to 29% of those in Social Class I, the professionals.[4] The general practitioners came at the same time as the consultant on rather less than half, 46%, of the domiciliary consultations.

Most of the general practitioners obviously appreciated the possibility of organising domiciliary consultations. Nearly all, 95%, thought the arrangements for them satisfactory.

> 'Very satisfactory—usually within 48 hours, frequently the same day—depending on the acuteness of the illness.'

[1] See Cartwright, Ann, *Human Relations and Hospital Care*, p. 28.

[2] G.P. Question 7: 'Could you estimate how many domiciliary consultations you have asked for in the last twelve months for patients with terminal illness?'

[3] Patients in hospital or institution all the year have been excluded.

[4] The classification used is based on the General Register Office's *Classification of Occupations* (1966). The information about the person's occupation, or for married or widowed women their husband's occupation, was obtained from the death certificate. See Appendix IV.

TABLE 39 *Difficulty in arranging admission and number of domiciliary consultations*

Estimated number of domiciliary consultations in last twelve months for patients with terminal illness	*Score of difficulty in arranging admission* 0 or 1	2	3	4 or 5	6+	*All general practitioners*
	%	%	%	%	%	%
None	52	43	25	26	27	32
1–4	35	41	59	47	44	46
5+	13	16	16	27	29	22
Number of general practitioners (=100%)	31	44	51	113	66	305

But there were some difficulties and criticism.

> 'Rarely used because of the difficulty in arranging contact with a specialist—they are not always gracious about accepting such a consultation.'

> 'No difficulty in getting them done. I would like to be present but often the consultant pops in on his own—won't agree to a time with me. I think it would be more satisfactory if we saw the patient together.'

> 'This domiciliary consultation is really a farce. It is merely a method of getting people into hospital and short-circuiting out-patients.'

General practitioners did not appear anxious just to pass on responsibility for a group of patients needing a lot of care, as many of them expressed a desire for direct access to N.H.S. beds which they could use for terminally ill patients and retain full responsibility for their treatment. A quarter said they had direct access to some N.H.S. beds where they retained full responsibility for treatment of their patients while in hospital, and most of these, a fifth of all general practitioners, said they could use some of the beds for patients in terminal care. Seventy-one per cent of those who had not got such beds said they would like some; and of those who had them, 85% said they would like more.

Nearly half the general practitioners, 48%, thought that if they had more time it would be appropriate for them to look after more patients who were terminally ill at home, and this proportion was 67% among those who felt that they were not able to give enough time to patients in terminal care and would like to give more time. Altogether two-fifths felt they would like to give more time to these patients, three-fifths that they gave enough time. But, as one doctor put it, 'The amount of time required is hard to define. Obviously one could usefully spend much more time as a "guide, philosopher and friend" especially with their emotional problems—but such time can never be adequately available until there is one doctor to one patient.' And many of the doctors who thought it would be appropriate for them to look after more terminally ill patients at home if they had more time qualified this: 'but there would have to be supporting services'. Those who felt it would not be appropriate to look after more terminally ill patients varied from many who thought they 'already looked after all those who could be looked after at home' to a few who thought it not generally appropriate to do so anyway: 'most relatives, I find, want their dying kinfolk in hospital'.

One general practitioner in our pilot study said that no expected deaths should be allowed to happen at home. We asked the general practitioners in the main inquiry whether they agreed or disagreed with this. The great majority, 94%, disagreed, but 6% agreed. Are the ones who agreed newly qualified doctors who would have little experience of death at home and might feel that the hospital was the only appropriate place for serious illness? On the contrary, none of those who agreed was under 45. The majority of the doctors who felt this were in single-handed practices or in a partnership with one other doctor (67% compared with 40% of those who disagreed). This supports a theory put forward in an earlier study that somewhat unusual practices—or in this instance exceptional views—are concentrated in single-handed or two-doctor practices.[1]

While only 15% of the general practitioners were critical about consultation with medical staff on the admission of patients, 60% were critical about consultations over discharge.

[1] Cartwright, Ann, *Parents and Family Planning Services*, p. 87.

In the last chapter we saw that the people who died at home after discharge from hospital had many symptoms and needed a lot of care. Inadequate consultation with general practitioners over the discharge of such patients will delay mobilisation of supporting community services. Comments from the general practitioners about the inadequacy of consultation over discharge ranged from statements about its complete non-existence—

> 'There is no contact whatsoever concerning the discharge of a patient—too often the relative informs you and then one has to await a discharge letter or contact the hospital.'

> 'Unfortunately we very often don't get discharge notes or anything to tell us they're out. Nobody goes and assesses the home condition.'

to complaints about delays—

> 'Letters reach us about a patient's discharge three days or a week later—I've known it to be a month. Relatives come to me and say "You've not been to see Auntie Jo since she came out of hospital". I have to tell them I've not received news of her discharge. It should be possible for housemen to sign letters and see they are posted when they do their rounds each day.'

about the inadequacy of the contents of discharge notes—

> 'Junior or nursing staff write discharge notes—very inadequate—just a little note—no treatment notes or what pills he's been having.'

and about the lack of suitable arrangements—

> 'The occasional unexpected discharge to unsuitable home conditions causes a great deal of difficulty.'

This sort of inadequate communication between hospitals and general practitioners is not likely to facilitate a good relationship between general practitioners and patients' relatives. A study by Brocklehurst and Shergold in which they interviewed geriatric patients who had been discharged from hospital also revealed that there was 'the need for bridges between home and hospital'.[1]

Relatives and general practitioners

The general practitioner can give help and support to those looking after people who are ill and frail at home. We asked the people we interviewed if they had the same doctor as the person who died and if not whether they knew the person's doctor at all. Seven-tenths had the same doctor or a different doctor in the same partnership, another fifth knew the dead person's doctor, leaving one in ten who had not known him. (The proportion with the same doctor was much higher for husbands and wives, 85%, than for other relatives, 56%, or friends and neighbours, 28%.) Those who knew the dead person's general practitioner were asked if they thought the doctor was an easy person to talk to or not. Most, 75%, thought he was easy, 14% said he was not, 11% were uncertain or made qualified comments. Many were enthusiastic:

> 'He was excellent—very wonderful. They both were. You could confide in them like one of yourselves.'
>
> 'You can ask him anything and he explains in simple language—he's marvellous.'
>
> 'He's a dear—one of the nicest men I ever met. I don't know a man I like as well as I like him.'

A number of those who were critical tried to explain their doctor's shortcomings:

> 'He could lose his temper but he could be kind too. He said once: "I don't know why you sent for me." But I expect he had a lot of people to see to. I can talk to the lady doctor better. She's a partner.'
>
> 'Some people find him very easy. I don't. I like him very much and get on well with his wife but I don't find him very easy. Someone said it was worse for him because he

[1] Brocklehurst, J. C. and Shergold, Margaret, 'What happens when geriatric patients leave hospital?'

knew he couldn't do anything. I don't think doctors ever really get used to losing patients.'

'He's rather an odd person. He's shy and he was born under Virgo and he's a perfectionist and a clinical man. He was very kind but it's an intellectual kindness rather than emotional. The ones under Pisces are more emotional.'

But some seemed to have an unsatisfactory relationship and were also critical when we asked whether they thought the doctor had time to discuss things or not.

'He doesn't give you a chance to explain things and at times he is very rude. He shouts at the poor old dears in the surgery and sends them away in tears.'

'He was not interested in my father—too much trouble. When I went down for a tonic for myself he seemed to think I was making too much of things. He never gave us the opportunity to discuss anything.'

Altogether 69% said the doctor had time to discuss things, 16% that he had not and 15% gave qualified answers as did a woman whose father-in-law had died of stomach cancer. He had come to live with them and became very weak in the last three months of his life, needing 'help with most things'. She found the general practitioner 'wasn't helpful. The problem arose because we thought he should be in hospital and the doctor said the only place he could get him in was a termination hospital. Of course we didn't want that. Then the doctor was quite off-hand and just shrugged his shoulders.'

Finding it easy to talk to a general practitioner was highly correlated with the view that he had time to discuss things. Eighty-four per cent of those who said he was easy to talk to thought he had time to discuss things, as did 8% of those who said he was not easy to talk to and 46% of the intermediate group. Altogether 64% thought he was both easy to talk to and had time to discuss things, 10% thought he had neither characteristic. One description of how the two were interrelated was:

'If there's something to discuss he'll sit and talk and you'll feel that you're the only person in the surgery and he has all the time in the world.'

The more often the person who died had consulted the general practitioner in the last year of life the more likely was the person we interviewed to have a good opinion of him. The proportion who thought he was both easy to talk to and had time to discuss things rose from 46% when the person who died had seen him once to 73% when he had seen him twenty or more times, while the proportion who were critical on both scores fell from 19% to 3%. This relationship could arise in two ways: the more care the doctor gave the people who died the more highly their relatives thought of him, but it is also possible that people who did not have a good relationship with their doctors were less likely to consult him. Two studies have shown that the frequency with which patients consult their doctors was related to doctors' views about the proportion of consultations they felt were either trivial, unnecessary or inappropriate[1] or for ailments that people could treat or cope with themselves without seeing the doctor.[2] This suggests that some doctors have, either deliberately or unconsciously, an off-putting or discouraging manner which makes patients hesitant about consulting them.

Further confirmation of this technique of discouragement, or lack of understanding, between doctors and patients comes from one of the questions we asked the general practitioners: 'On the whole do you find in this area that most relatives accept reasonable responsibility for home care or do they seek admission to hospital or institution?' A third thought most accepted responsibility, a quarter that most sought admission to a hospital or institution for their relatives, the rest that it was equally balanced. The doctors who thought that most accepted responsibility apparently gave more care to patients who were dying than the doctors who were rather critical of relatives. Thirty-eight per cent of the patients whose doctor thought most relatives accepted responsibility had twenty or more consultations in the year before they died, 25% of the others. Doctors who visit patients frequently may be more aware of the amount of care given by relatives and the burden this involves. (Thirty-one per cent of the patients whose doctor thought

[1] Cartwright, Ann, *Patients and their Doctors*, p. 51.

[2] Dunnell, Karen and Cartwright, Ann, *Medicine Takers, Prescribers and Hoarders*, pp. 66–7.

most relatives accepted responsibility had 20 or more home visits in the year compared with 21% of the others.) There were no clear differences in the proportions dying at home or in hospital between patients whose doctors had different views on the care given by relatives.

But when doctors felt relatives were reluctant to look after patients they reported more difficulty in obtaining admissions. (Their average score on difficulty of obtaining admissions was 4·7 compared with 3·7 of those who thought most relatives accepted responsibility and 4·0 for the intermediate group.)

Doctors who experience much difficulty in making suitable arrangements for the care of their patients may feel frustrated and more apt to blame relatives. Their expectations and earlier experiences may also colour their reactions. The proportion who felt most relatives sought admission rose from 12% of the doctors under 40 to 27% of those between 40 and 60, and 33% of those aged 60 or more. But relatives' views on whether the doctor was easy to talk to or had time to discuss things were unrelated to the doctor's age or his opinions about the willingness of people to look after their dying relations.[1]

The general practitioner and community services

When the person who died had been helped by people from the local health authority it was the general practitioner who generally arranged it. The proportions were 91% of those receiving care from a district nurse, 68% of those who had had a home help and 65% of those who had been visited by a health visitor. The general practitioner had also played a part in making the arrangement for 53% of those who had other nursing care at home, 21% of those seen by a chiropodist and 17% of those helped by others such as the association for the physically handicapped, the welfare officer for the blind and officers from the Department of Health and Social Security. Obviously the general practitioner plays a key role in the distribution of community care. What do the doctors think about these services in their areas?

[1] The three factors shown to be associated with doctors' feelings about relatives' desire for hospital admission—the doctor's age, his views on the difficulty of obtaining hospital admission, and the frequency with which patients with terminal illness consulted him—were not related to each other.

A quarter regarded the home help service in their areas as adequate, half thought it 'rather inadequate', the other quarter as 'very inadequate'.[1] Just over a half, 55%, thought more home help services were needed in their areas and one in ten thought this more urgent than additional hospital beds.

A quarter thought more district nurses were needed in their areas, but few, less than one in twenty, felt this was more important than other needs.[2] In general they were appreciative of the care given by district nurses: 85% thought the service 'very helpful' for patients at home with terminal illness, the other 15% thought it 'moderately helpful', none (that is less than 1%) said it was not helpful.

General practitioners were less enthusiastic about the help given by health visitors to patients at home with terminal illness. A quarter regarded them as 'very helpful', a quarter as 'moderately helpful' and half as 'not helpful'. But this may just reflect the fact that many health visitors are not involved in the care of dying patients.

We asked general practitioners about their use and views of a number of other services which might be organised by local authorities or by voluntary associations. Replies are in Table 40.

The services most often judged to be inadequate were night sitting and night nursing services. Over two-fifths of the doctors in areas which had such services wanted them extended, and between two-thirds and three-quarters of the doctors in areas which did not have them would like them introduced. Even so it seems strange that when services did not exist so many general practitioners felt they were not needed—the proportion ranged from a quarter feeling this about night nursing services to half or more about a bathing service, the supply of sickroom equipment and a service for disposing of incontinence pads. They may have felt that the numbers were too small to justify such a service, but it may be that some of the general practitioners were unaware of the extent of the problems relatives faced in looking after people at home.

[1] In a study in six areas in 1965 three-fifths of the general practitioners interviewed thought home helps were the most urgently needed additional local health authority workers. Hockey, Lisbeth, *Feeling the Pulse*, p. 83.

[2] And in the same study mentioned in the previous footnote, over half the doctors considered that the district nursing service could advantageously be widened (p. xi).

TABLE 40 *General practitioners' use of and views on various community services*

	Meals on wheels	*Special laundry service*	*Free supply of incontinence pads*	*Service for disposing of incontinence pads*	*Bathing service*	*Supply of sickroom equipment*	*Night nursing service*	*Night sitting service*	*Geriatric social worker*
	%	%	%	%	%	%	%	%	%
Used	83	28	64	18	38	67	17	24	32
Not used but available	12	8	12	5	9	14	9	10	13
Not available	3	56	18	62	51	18	70	62	50
Don't know if available	2	8	6	15	2	1	4	4	5
Number of general practitioners (=100%)[a]					319				
Would like extended[b]	26% (301)	4% (112)	7% (241)	3% (72)	9% (149)	15% (256)	41% (82)	46% (108)	19% (142)
Would like introduced[c]	63% (16)	57% (200)	58% (76)	44% (245)	50% (167)	48% (61)	70% (234)	77% (209)	63% (173)

[a] Those for whom inadequate information was obtained have been omitted when calculating the percentages.
[b] Based on number saying service available.
[c] Based on number saying service not available or not knowing if available.

Other studies have found that general practitioners did not always know of the existence of services.[1] We found that the general practitioners in the different study areas did not always agree on whether or not a service was available in their area. (The extent of disagreement, from either 100% or 0%, averaged 19% for the nine services in the twelve areas.) Comparisons with the information obtained from the superintendents of

[1] Anderson, J. A. D. and Warren, Elizabeth A., 'Communications with general practitioners'; Gilhome, K. R. and Newell, D. J., 'Community services for the elderly'.

district nurses (and the superintendents of health visitors, if they were different people) showed that when the superintendents said a service existed on average 69% of the general practitioners said it was available; when the superintendents said it did not exist this average was 15%, and the average was 35% when the service was said to be available in part of the area or when there was conflicting information from two superintendents. Some general practitioners will of course have patients in other nearby areas and may be referring to the services there. And in large or widespread areas the existence of a service in one part of the area may not mean that it is effectively available in all parts, even of the same administrative district. Taking these limitations into account, the data suggest that general practitioners may often be unaware that services are available in their area—but sometimes services may be available in theory but very limited in practice. Occasionally, too, doctors may assume that services exist when they do not, or superintendents may be misinformed or unaware of some services—particularly, for example, if there is a geriatric social worker attached to a hospital.

Summary and conclusions

The general practitioner plays a key role in the care of the dying. He gave nearly all the medical care to about three-tenths of the people in our sample in the last year of their lives and he usually looked after the other seven-tenths before they were admitted to hospital and arranged for their admission. He made many visits to those who had been in hospital but came home to die. The patients with whom the general practitioner had frequent contact (twenty or more consultations in the year) had many symptoms. More of them than of the people dying in hospital were reported to suffer from bedsores, incontinence and trouble with breathing. So when nearly nine-tenths of general practitioners said they had difficulty in making suitable arrangements under the National Health Service for elderly patients needing long-term nursing care this indicates a deficiency in the service which must lead to much suffering and discomfort for patients and place a heavy burden on their relatives and friends who look after them. This deficiency has been revealed by other studies[1] and shows the impotence of general practitioners to campaign effectively for the services their patients need. General practitioners do not seem to want, or feel it is inappropriate for them, to act as a pressure group to improve services. And while they were aware of inadequacies in the availability of certain types of in-patient care they seemed much less aware of deficiencies in various forms of community care. A number were complacent about non-existent community services.[2]

Failure to recognise needs for community services which can help relatives and friends in the care of patients at home suggests that general practitioners do not give as much support as they might to caring relatives, nor do the doctors always seem to appreciate the amount of care that relatives and friends provide, or the extent and full nature of patients' needs in the last year of their lives. One of the most disturbing findings was the high proportion of people with symptoms who had not sought the help of their doctor—or of anyone else. The data suggest that this stems partly from a realistic assessment of the inability of the profession to help with some problems, but partly from anxiety or fear and partly because some felt that their general practitioner had not time to discuss things, some people were not seeking help for symptoms which probably could have been relieved.

[1] Cartwright, Ann, *Human Relations and Hospital Care*, pp. 23–6.

[2] Other studies have found general practitioners more complacent than health visitors about family planning services (Cartwright, Ann, *Parents and Family Planning Services*, p. 165) and less aware than district nurses of the need for home help services (Hockey, Lisbeth, *Feeling the Pulse*, p. 83).

6

THE DISTRICT NURSE

A third of the people who died and who had been at home for some time during the year before their death had been helped by a district nurse during this time. In this chapter we describe the frequency and nature of this help, who received it, the relationship between district nurses and general practitioners and other services, and the views of district nurses.

Frequency and amount of care

Much of the care given by district nurses was of a comparatively short-term nature—presumably during a crisis before the person died or was admitted to hospital. Half had been helped for less than a month, including a fifth who had her help for less than a week.[1] A fifth had been helped for between one and three months, three-tenths for more than three months including one in seven (that is one in twenty of all those who died[2]) who had help for a year or longer. The numbers and frequency of consultations are shown in Table 41. Relatively few, just over two-fifths, of those who had long-term help for a year or more ever had daily help.

The district nurse was more likely to have helped when the person needed short-term rather than long-term care. For instance when the person who died had needed help with washing or shaving the district nurse had helped 37% of those needing such help for less than a year compared with 22% of those who needed it for longer; comparable proportions for those who had to be given a bedpan or bottle were 23% and 9% and for those needing help with bandaging or dressing 71% and 48%. Nearly a quarter of the people who died, 23%,

[1] This is based on data from the relatives: Question 52b: 'For how long did he have that sort of help?'

[2] Excluding those in a hospital or institution for the year.

TABLE 41 *Number and frequency of district nurse visits (data from relatives)*

	Period over which received help					
	Less than a week	*A week but less than a month*	*One month but less than three months*	*Three months but less than a year*	*A year or more*	*All receiving help*
Number of visits in last twelve months	%	%	%	%	%	%
1–2	73	2	—	—	3	16
3–5	18	10	4	6	—	8
6–11	9	27	7	3	3	12
12–19	—	31	16	6	9	15
20–49	—	30	39	28	9	21
50–299	—	—	34	57	47	23
300+	—	—	—	—	29	5
How often (at most frequent)[a]	%	%	%	%	%	%
Daily	22	79	65	62	43	56
Less than daily—weekly	6	21	28	29	36	23
Less than weekly	72[b]	—	7	9	21	21
Number of deaths (=100%)[c]	48	65	46	35	35	234

[a] Question 52c: 'How often did he have that sort of help—at its most frequent?'
[b] Includes those with a single visit.
[c] Those for whom inadequate information was obtained have been excluded when calculating percentages.

were felt to have needed help from a district nurse more often[1] and this proportion was nearly half, 46%, for those who had been visited only once or twice.

Some comments from relatives were:

> 'The one visit a day was helpful but I had to wash and change him half a dozen times a day.' (Daughter whose father had been semi-paralysed for over a year and doubly incontinent for more than three months. She had asked the general practitioner about having more help, but 'he seemed to think I had enough help'.)

[1] Question 52e: 'Do you feel he had that help as often as necessary or would it have been better if he'd had it more or less often?'

One daughter whose mother had daily visits from district nurses for ten days for injections would have liked them to visit longer but said: 'Some aren't as helpful as others. One used to wash her down a bit.'

No one felt the district nurse had visited too often. A fifth would have liked her to do other things besides the things she did do.

A wife aged 76 whose husband had been incontinent of urine for about two years and died of cancer had had a visit from a district nurse every three weeks for over a year to change his catheter and the nurse sometimes gave him an enema. But she would have liked more help, because 'I could have kept him at home then', for lifting and washing him. She'd asked the doctor about this and he said her husband must go into hospital. 'He [husband] was very averse to it. I carried on as long as I could. I had to coax him to go—it was awful.' He died four days after being admitted.

A daughter whose mother had died of sarcoma of the femur said the district nurse had helped with washing and lifting her mother but 'said she didn't do dressings. I think she was scared. But later I did get help from another nurse who came.'

But most of those who had wanted extra help, nearly two-thirds, had not asked anyone about the possibility: 'I just felt I had to cope.' About a third of those who had asked said there had been some change in the arrangements as a result.

Nature of care

The different types of help the district nurses were said to have given to patients are shown in Table 42. When people needed such nursing procedures as enemas, dressings or bandages, regular temperature-taking or injections the district nurse helped in nearly half or more instances. She also helped a third of those needing help with washing or shaving, a quarter of those needing lifting and a fifth of those who needed a bedpan or bottle. But the type of help she most often gave, shown in the second column, was with washing or shaving, lifting, dressings or injections.

When a person needing nursing care was visited by a district nurse she generally helped directly, except for giving medicines. Often she helped with personal care, too, but rarely with night care. Just over half the people visited by a district nurse were said to need care at night, but she helped only one out of

TABLE 42 *Types of help given by district nurse (data from relatives)*

	Proportion helped by district nurse		
	Of all those needing that type of help	*Of all those visited by district nurse*	*Of all those needing that type of help and visited*
He p needed at home with:			
Lifting	27% (342)	39%	47% (188)
Washing or shaving	34% (381)	54%	60% (210)
Getting in or out of bath	18% (215)	16%	35% (102)
Dressing or undressing	13% (295)	16%	24% (152)
Getting in or out of bed	12% (305)	16%	22% (167)
Getting hair washed at home	13% (258)	15%	23% (142)
Cutting toenails	16% (339)	23%	31% (171)
Giving bedpan or bottle	20% (173)	15%	32% (104)
Getting to lavatory or commode	13% (310)	17%	23% (167)
Any type of self care	32%	71%	[a]
Giving medicine or tablets	9% (315)	11%	15% (176)
Injections	47% (142)	29%	67% (100)
Bandaging or other dressing	65% (107)	29%	80% (84)
Regular temperature-taking	60% (31)	8%	72% (25)
Massaging/exercises	22% (91)	9%	44% (45)
Enema	90% (42)	15%	95% (38)
Other nursing procedure	52% (73)	16%	74% (51)
Any nursing procedure	40%	74%	[a]
Sitting up with at night	3% (217)	2%	4% (123)
Other help at night	3% (238)	3%	5% (129)
Any night care	3%	3%	[a]
Help with housework	1%	1%	[a]
Number of people visited by district nurses (=100%)	234		

The figures in brackets are the numbers on which the percentages are based (=100%)

[a] Figures not available as these analyses were done on the particular items with which help was needed.

twenty of these. This does not mean that the other people did not get help when they needed it. Data in Chapter 2 showed that wives, husbands and daughters were the most common sources of help for many types of care.

So far the type of care and its frequency have been looked at from the data given to us by relatives of the deceased. But we also have some information from the district nurses about the care given to some of the patients in our sample. The district nurses we interviewed identified 179 of our sample of 960 deaths as people to whom they had given some care in their homes. Comparison of the information received from nurses and relatives suggests that relatives forgot or were unaware that the nurse had visited in about 5% where a nurse helped and they failed to identify the district nurse as such in another 3%.[1] The nurses identified about 54% of the people reported by relatives to have received some care. We thought that the nurses might be more likely to recall and identify patients they visited on several occasions than they would those they saw only once or twice. Comparison with the information from the relatives confirmed this. They reported twenty or more visits from a district nurse for 57% of the patients recalled by the nurses and 40% of the others, while the proportion with only one or two visits was 12% of the 'matched' cases, 22% of the 'unmatched'. So the 'sample' on which the nurses reported seems to have been a biased one.

Certainly the data from the nurses suggest they gave rather more intensive care than was reported by relatives. They said that 40% of the patients they identified had fifty or more visits from a district nurse in the last twelve months of their lives. Relatives reported that, of the people they identified as having district nurse care, 28% had as many visits. (The correlation between the number of visits reported by relatives and nurses for the 'matched' patients was 0·61.)

[1] For thirty-one of the people identified by district nurses as receiving some help—17% of those they identified—we did not obtain an interview. In four instances the district nurse was described as 'another nurse' and in another as 'a friend who was also a district nurse'. In the remaining 143 instances the data from the two sources 'matched' for 127 (89%) the nurse appeared to have recalled a different person in five, the relative to have forgotten or to have been unaware that the person had been helped in seven and there were various other discrepancies or confusions over the other four.

The help the nurses reported they gave to the 179 patients they identified is shown in Table 43. The figures in the left half of the table can be compared with those in the middle column of the previous table. Nurses reported giving more of all the types of help listed there except for bandaging or dressing and help getting in or out of the bath. The more technical nursing procedures are listed on the right hand side of the table. Washing or shaving, bedmaking, the care of pressure areas, and the taking of temperature, pulse and respiration

TABLE 43 *Help reported by district nurses*

	%		%
Lifting	72	Lavage/douche/pessary	11
Washing or shaving	83	Catheterisation	3
Getting in or out of bath	16	Blood pressure	2
Dressing or undressing	34	Eye/ear drops	2
Getting in or out of bed	59	Care of pressure areas	79
Getting hair washed at home	23	Electrocardiogram	1
Cutting toenails	57	Dialysis	—
Giving bedpan or bottle	48	Taking temperature, pulse, respiration	73
Getting to lavatory or commode	42	Other nursing procedures	13
Bed-making	80	None of these	13
None of these	7		
	%		%
Giving medicines or tablets	32	Teaching patient self care	26
Injections	35	Teaching relatives	53
Bandaging or other dressing	29	Supervision only	20
Regular temperature-taking for hypothermia prevention	14	None of these	33
Massaging/exercises	25		
Enema	21		
None of these	21		

Number of patients in sample identified by nurses and visited at home (=100%) 179[a]

[a] Small numbers for whom inadequate information was obtained have been omitted when calculating percentages.

rates were each recorded for about three-quarters of the patients visited.

Further evidence of the intensity of care reported by the nurses is that 25% of their patients were said to have been visited at night (between 8 p.m. and 8 a.m.), and 48% to have had more than seven visits in a single week.[1] The most usual amount of time they spent on a visit was between thirty and forty-five minutes. The distribution is shown in Table 44.

TABLE 44 *Time district nurses estimated they spent on visits*

	Usually	*At most*	*At least*
	%	%	%
Less than 10 minutes	1	1	7
10 minutes but less than 20	13	7	29
20 minutes but less than 30	23	9	35
30 minutes but less than 45	37	23	18
45 minutes but less than 1 hour	17	29	6
1 hour but less than 1½ hours	8	26	5
1½ hours or more	1	5	—
Number of patients in sample identified by nurses (=100%)	171		

Whom did the district nurse help?[2]

Women were more likely to have been helped by a district nurse than men (41% compared with 27%), people aged 75 or over more than younger people (47% compared with 25%), and those with cancer more than those dying from other diseases (45% compared with 28%).[3]

District nurses were also more likely to have helped those who died at home than those dying in a hospital or institution, 45% against 24%. But, as we saw in Chapter 4, over half, 53%, of those who had been in hospital at some time during the

[1] Question 12: 'Is it possible to say from the records what was the maximum number of visits —— had during any one week—I mean visits at any time of the day?'

[2] People who were in a hospital or institution for all the twelve months before they died have been omitted from this section.

[3] Age, sex and cause of death are all related, but each was related, independently, to help from the district nurse.

year but had died at home had been visited by a district nurse, as opposed to 35% of others dying at home.

In some ways the district nurse compensated for the absence of a spouse. This is suggested by the differences with marital status and household composition shown in Table 45. Those who were widowed and those living with relatives but not a spouse were the ones most likely to have been helped.

TABLE 45 *Marital status, household composition and help from a district nurse*

	Percentage helped by a district nurse	*Number of deaths (=100%)*
Marital status		
Single	33%	70
Married	29%	386
Widowed or divorced	42%	235
Household composition		
On own	21%	99
With spouse with or without others of same or older generation	28%	234
With spouse and others of a younger generation	29%	150
With relatives of same or older generation only	48%	40
With relatives of younger generation	51%	156
With unrelated people or in guesthouses	21%	24

Relatively few people living on their own had been helped by a district nurse, but this was partly at any rate because they had few restrictions and district-nurse care was strongly related to the extent of restriction. The proportion who had been visited by a district nurse declined from nine-tenths of those who had been bedridden for a year or more to one in fifty of those reported to have no restrictions.

The symptoms most clearly related to district-nurse care were bedsores (72% of the people with this had been visited by a district nurse), unpleasant smell (59%), incontinence (56%), and mental confusion (51%).

These findings seem rather different to those described in the previous chapter. There it was reported that only 7% of the patients with an unpleasant smell had sought the advice of a district nurse about it and 58% had not sought advice from anyone. The district nurse may have cared and helped but she was not seen as a source of advice.

Help from a district nurse was nearly always arranged by a general practitioner, and the two types of help were clearly related. The proportion visited by a district nurse rose from 10% of those with less than five general practitioner consultations in the year to 56% of those with twenty or more. Obviously communication between district nurses and general practitioners is important for arranging appropriate and effective help. Their relationship is discussed next.

The relationship between district nurses and general practitioners

Half the doctors said they had a district nurse attached to their practice, and those who did were more appreciative of her services, less likely to want any changes in the service or the way it was organised, and more likely to ask her to visit when the patient just needed care that relatives were able and willing to give.[1] This is shown in Table 46.

A number of those wanting changes in the service or its organisation sought attachments or a closer relationship between the nurses and the general practitioners.

> 'I'd like to see more of a tie up with G.P.s. These practices which have a district nurse attached must be better than practices where you don't meet one another and all consultations are over the phone.'

Others wanted a rather different involvement:

> 'More authority given to G.P.s so as to use district nurses to maximum benefit.'

Several wanted more nurses:

> 'An increase in the number of district nurses so that the nurses can spend more time with their patients.'

[1] G.P. Question 14: 'If a patient needs just nursing care that relatives are able and prepared to give do you tend to ask the district nurse to visit or not?'

TABLE 46 *General practitioners' views of the district nursing services, for those with and without a district nurse attached to their practice*

	General practitioners:		
Practitioners' views	*With a district nurse attached*	*Without a district nurse attached*	*All general practitioners*
For patients at home with terminal illness find the district nursing service:	%	%	%
Very helpful	92	78	85
Moderately helpful	8	21	15
Not helpful	—	1	—
Would like some changes in the service or its organisation	33%	44%	38%
Would like them to give other sorts of help or care	10%	19%	15%
Tends to ask the district nurse to visit when patient needs just care that relatives are able and prepared to give	52%	33%	43%
Number of general practitioners (=100%)[a]	160	160	323

[a] Those for whom inadequate information was obtained have been excluded when the percentages were calculated.

Other suggestions were:

> 'More part-timers could be employed to provide full-time day care [nine to five] for the last week of terminal cases. This would be much cheaper than using a hospital bed and very acceptable to elderly couples. Many married nurses would welcome a chance for temporary work.'

> 'Should perhaps have more assistant nurses to do routine things—baths, etc. S.R.N.s are wasted on simple jobs.'

> 'Perhaps it should be possible for nurses to visit patients more frequently over weekends and at night.'

Night services were also mentioned as an additional type of help the doctors would like the nurses or someone to give:

> 'I would like to have the occasional use of night nursing and sitting services.'

> 'If we could have some system where someone could help families at night to give them a rest—but whether this should be district nurses or not I don't know.'

Comments from those who tended to ask the nurse to visit when the patient needed just nursing care that the relatives were able and willing to give were:

> 'Her expert help and guidance with nursing procedure is appreciated, gives the relatives reassurance that they are doing the job correctly, and while she is in the house there is a short rest from responsibility.'

> 'If it's a terminal illness sooner or later they are going to need at least moral support. Also the district nurse is able to give advice.'

When doctors asked nurses to visit at this early stage more of their patients who died had been visited by a district nurse—48% compared with 32% of the patients whose doctor did not ask at that stage.

A few district nurses, 4%, felt general practitioners tended to ask for district nursing help earlier than necessary; more, 14%, felt they did not ask for it early enough. Comments illustrating this last view were:

> 'We don't get called until they have bedsores. Doctors always think we are too busy and if the patients are dying already it doesn't matter. I'd like to go earlier.'

> 'They usually send for you about two days before they go into hospital. They expect relatives to do things they don't or can't.'

> 'I feel there are some cases where they are in the very last stages—bedsores, incontinence, etc. If we had been called in earlier perhaps these things could be avoided. Probably because they think this is an incurable case from a medical

point of view there's not much anybody can do. But we as district nurses can help a lot.'

Some examples they gave about this were:

> 'A little old lady with cardiac. Going past her cottage one morning I was flagged down by the person living with her. She'd fallen down and had sores and bruises on her back and had been in bed all summer.'

> 'A man with gangrene of the feet had been home indefinitely. If we'd been called in earlier we could have prevented bedsores with the use of a ripple bed. It's partly that the doctors feel we have enough on and they're reluctant to add to our over-strained system.'

One nurse who was attached to a practice and felt that general practitioners asked at the right time described the relationship this created:

> 'I am usually sent in to begin with to build up a friendship and get to know the patient, and build up from there. Then you can assess what is necessary for the nursing care and patients by that time have gained something by your early visits. I feel our early visits are very important to the patient, to be able to talk to them and answer their questions and give them confidence although yourself you know they are terminally ill. I feel it's very important to brighten the darkness for them—not just to rush in, take your coat off and start doing things for them. If it's a slow but sure ending I think it's important to spend as much time as possible with the patient and give moral support to the relatives as well.'

A comment from one who thought she was called in earlier than necessary shows that the nurses themselves, like the general practitioners, vary in their conception of their role. She was apparently complaining when she said: 'I think sometimes they send you for moral support'.

Table 47 shows that nurses who were attached to a general medical practice were less likely to feel that general practitioners did not refer patients early enough, and relatively few of them—a tenth compared with a quarter of nurses not attached to a practice—regarded their contact with general practitioners over patients with a terminal illness as inadequate. But less than half the nurses thought the information they were given when patients were referred was generally adequate and, although this proportion was slightly greater for the attached nurses, clearly attachment does not solve this problem.

TABLE 47 *District nurses' views of their relationships with general practitioners for those attached and those not attached to a general practice*

	District nurses		
District nurses' views	*Attached to a general practice*	*Not attached to a general practice*	*All district nurses*
Find that on the whole for patients with terminal illness general practitioners ask for district nursing help:	%	%	%
Earlier than necessary	4	4	4
Not early enough	8	23	15
About right time	81	61	72
Qualified answer	7	12	9
In caring for patients in terminal illness feel contact with general practitioner is generally:	%	%	%
Adequate	88	72	81
Rather inadequate	8	21	14
Very inadequate	1	4	2
Qualified answer	3	3	3
On referral of patients for district nursing care thinks information given is generally:	%	%	%
Adequate	46	34	42
Rather inadequate	36	41	38
Very inadequate	13	16	14
Qualified answer	5	9	6
Number of district nurses (=100%)[a]	281	225	506

[a] A small number for whom inadequate information was obtained have been excluded when the percentages were calculated.

Looking now at the nurses' relationships with individual patients in our sample: two-fifths of the requests to visit were made by personal contact. This proportion was 58% when the nurse was attached to a general practice, 28% when she was not. The nurse regarded the information she was given about the individual patients as adequate in 82% of the cases. This proportion was 90% when she had direct personal contact with the person making the request, 78% when it was made by the person over the telephone and 72% when she received a letter or message.

Although nurses attached to general practices appeared to have a more satisfactory relationship with their general practitioner colleagues they were even more critical than other nurses of their contact with hospitals. The proportion who regarded it as adequate was 27% among attached nurses, 38% among unattached. Does their closer contact with general practitioners make them less able to maintain or develop contact with hospitals or just more critical of the inadequacy of present arrangements? This is one of many questions raised but not answered by this study.

A possible indication of the effect of district nurse attachments to general practitioners was that 42% of the people who died[1] whose doctor had a district nurse attached to his practice had been visited by a district nurse compared with 28% of those whose doctor did not have such an attachment. But unfortunately we do not have information about the caseloads of nurses working in these different situations.

Views of the district nurses

Like the general practitioners, most of the district nurses, 96%, disagreed with the doctor who said that no anticipated deaths should be allowed to happen at home. Several took almost the opposite view: 'Home is the natural place to die in. People need to be among their own friends and relatives not among strangers.' 'Everybody prefers to die in their own homes with their families and familiar things around them.' But this comment seems to sum up the view of the majority:

> 'I think it depends on the circumstances. Each case must be viewed on its merits. Some people are horrified at the thought of having to care for the dying—they are nervous

[1] Excluding those who had been in a hospital or other institution for a year or more and those who died unexpectedly.

and need support. Others prefer to care for their own relatives and are capable of doing it. I don't think anyone should be persuaded to go into hospital against their will or the will of their relatives.'

Nearly two-thirds of the district nurses felt that they would like to give more time to patients in terminal illness but just over a third felt that on the whole they were able to give enough time to these patients.[1] A quarter thought more time was needed for additional nursing care.

> 'People with bedsores need to be turned more often and incontinents dried. It's often not done from one visit to the next—when I go again.'

> 'I'd like to give them more nursing care and to be able to extend all the things we do—a better wash, more change of clothing. Could do with going in in twos so they could be lifted out and the bed made properly.'

Over two-fifths, 44%, wished their visits were not so rushed so that there would be more time 'to chat with the patient to make it more on a friendly basis. At the moment we have to rush in and do our work and rush out. If you chat to them it reassures them.'

> 'So often elderly people especially like you to sit and talk to them. There is always the thought at the back of your mind "I must get on". If you had more time to sit and talk they would tell you more of their problems.'

> 'For people living on their own who just have odd relatives going in, it seems to help them if they unload their burdens to us. They feel as though somebody is listening who cares for them.'

Several mentioned their desire to spend more time with relatives.

> 'To reassure the relatives that they are doing all they can. Supportive for them. To become not just a nurse—you want to become their friend.'

[1] Nurses' question 11: 'On the whole do you feel you are able to give enough time to patients in terminal illness or would you like to be able to give more time to them?'

'To reassure the family and to teach people how to help the patient in your absence. This takes a great deal of time.'

At the same time four-fifths of the nurses regarded the district nursing service for patients in terminal illness in their area as 'adequate'; only one in a hundred thought it 'very inadequate', the others thought it 'rather inadequate'. A number of those who described it as adequate added qualifications—'as long as we are willing to work ourselves to death'. 'We could do with more staff. If we had more bath attendants we could give more time to ill patients who need us.' And the point that more bath attendants, state enrolled nurses and supporting services would give the district nurses more scope was also made by a number of those who thought the present service rather inadequate. When asked about the particular patients in our sample, they felt they gave enough time to about three-quarters but would have liked to give more time to the other quarter.

District nurses were less likely than general practitioners to feel that most relatives sought admission to hospital rather than accepting responsibility for home care: 9% compared with 25%. In general they were visiting more frequently than doctors so they were likely to be more aware of all the care given by relatives and the burden this places on them. On the other hand, the views of general practitioners were based on all the patients they saw, which included some who were admitted to hospital and had never been seen by a district nurse.

Fewer nurses than general practitioners—33% against 51%—thought that 'unwillingness of relatives to look after them' was the main thing preventing more people being looked after in the community rather than in hospital. The nurses also seemed more aware of community services than general practitioners.

The district nurse and community services

Most district nurses said they had used the various community services we asked about if they were available (see Table 48). The existing services they were least likely to have used were night nursing and night sitting services and the geriatric social worker. When there was no special laundry service, bathing service or night service available in their area about three-quarters of the nurses said they would like one introduced; the other quarter apparently did not feel there was a need for them. Fewer, but still half or more, would have liked a geriatric social worker and a service for disposing of incontinence pads when one did not exist.

Their reports about the availability of services related fairly closely to the information given to us by nursing superintendents in the study areas. When a superintendent said a service existed, on average 88% of the district nurses said it was available (compared with 69% of general practitioners). Communications about local authority services are likely to be easier and more direct for the district nurses than the general practitioners. And the nurses, unlike the doctors, usually work within a single local authority health service area, so this question about services in their areas was more clearly defined for them.

On the whole, district nurses seemed better informed about various services and made more use of them than general practitioners. The nurses were also less complaisant about most of the existing services; they were more likely than the doctors to want meals on wheels, special laundry service, supply of incontinence pads, and a bathing service extended if they already existed or introduced if they did not. Altogether a third of the nurses said they would like to see some changes in the services discussed so far. Some suggestions were: better equipment (e.g. 'ripple beds for terminal cancers'), the laundry service extended ('to cover personal washing like nightwear and towels'), and the bathing service extended ('so that we can give more care to the very ill and the elderly'). A number said they would like services to be free or the costs reduced:

> 'The night nursing and sitting services are too expensive for some people. We should be allowed to use our discretion—and this also goes for the laundry service. It should be free to some people who just can't afford it.'

> 'I would like the night nursing and night sitting services to be provided by the County so people don't have to pay extortionate prices.'

TABLE 48 *The district nurse and community services*

	Meals on wheels	*Special laundry service*	*Supply of incontinence pads*[a]	*Service for disposing of incontinence pads*	*Bathing service*	*Supply of sickroom equipment*	*Night nursing service*	*Night sitting service*	*Geriatric social worker*
	%	%	%	%	%	%	%	%	%
Used	93	56	95	51	58	97	54	59	61
Not used but available	5	3	4	7	3	3	12	12	16
Not available	2	41	1	40	39	—	33	28	19
Not known if available	—	—	—	2	—	—	1	1	4
Number of district nurses (=100%)	506								
Would like extended[b]	65% (493)	19% (297)	17% (499)	12% (294)	55% (310)	16% (503)	43% (336)	57% (357)	15% (391)
Would like introduced[c]	82%[d] (11)	76% (204)	—	50% (201)	77% (194)	—	71% (165)	75% (142)	56% (97)

Figures in brackets are the numbers on which the percentages are based (=100%)

[a] The initial question was about the free supply of incontinence pads, but 61 district nurses, all in Birmingham, said there was a service in their area but it was not entirely free.

[b] Based on number saying the service was available.

[c] Based on number saying the service was not available.

[d] Based on less than 20 cases.

Two-fifths of the nurses thought there were other services which would be helpful in the care of terminally ill patients. Many of their suggestions were concerned with the help and support of relatives by day sitters or others.

> 'I think a day sitter, when there's a man and wife and no relatives, a day sitter to stay with the patient so that shopping and so on could be done would be a great help'.

> 'It would keep a lot of people out of hospital if relatives got more help than they do, even if it's only one night a week to go to the pictures.'

> 'Somebody who could just *sit* to give a relative a break during the day.'

> 'A visiting service would be helpful, mainly to sit with patients and to do the little odd jobs. I very often meet the problem of the relatives who are so housebound. I find that they are terribly housebound and they haven't always got help from outside, and the patients sort of get a clinging dependency on these relatives. That's why I think a visiting service of some kind.'

A number mentioned the need for financial help:

> 'I'd like to see some of the families having an allowance for the last few months so they can buy extras'.

> 'It would be a help if we could have free prescriptions for some patients who need a lot of tablets and drugs and dressings.'

> 'A grant of some sort—where you get a husband a year or two younger than the wife near pensionable age and you find they have to pay for getting some of the services and they cannot afford it—also for the young patient with family responsibilities.'

Again the need for more help at night was raised by a number of nurses. Other suggestions were a shaving service for men, occupational therapists, physiotherapists, library facilities, hairdressing and barber services, a day room for the elderly where they could get together, domiciliary chiropody, some means of taking housebound people on outings and 'something in between home helps and district nurses—like an orderly or have home helps seconded to the district nurse service for daily use'.

The district nurse and the hospital

The often non-existent relationship between the district nurse and the hospital illustrates the disadvantage of the tripartite system in the National Health Service and the way in which individuals adapt to, accept, or manipulate administrative systems which seem to impede and restrict their effective co-operation.

When asked: 'In caring for patients in terminal illness do you feel contact with the hospital is generally adequate, rather inadequate or very inadequate?', one-third described it as adequate, one-third as rather inadequate, a quarter as very inadequate, and one in nine said there was no contact. But few in this last group seemed critical, they simply stated it as a fact: 'I've never had any contact with the hospital.' Those who described it as adequate varied from those who seemed to accept little contact as appropriate:

> 'We don't have any contact. You don't need much contact with them. They send patients home without hope. It's all quite adequate.'
>
> 'If it's terminal they can't do anything anyway.'

To those who in one way or another had some contact:

> 'In our practice the reports are sent to the doctor and we have access to them now that we're in group practice'.
>
> 'I've made it my practice always to go to the hospital ward if ever in doubt. I've never had any hesitation about going straight to the ward.'
>
> 'I know the local hospital pretty well: I know a lot of the staff and get in touch with them.'

Comments from those who were more critical were:

> 'We get no information at all. I have only had two letters

from a sister about a patient which was wonderful. It would be helpful if this could happen in every case' (rather inadequate).

'You don't even know what operations they've had—got to take relative's word. Don't know what course of treatment to follow, no directions given' (rather inadequate).

'The message is far too brief that we get from the Almoner. I would like more information on what has been done, the diagnosis and the treatment. There is another thing: I do not agree when they discharge an elderly person to an empty house with no heating or lighting and nothing been checked to see if it's all right' (very inadequate).

Ideas about ways in which changes in the relationship between hospitals and district nurses could facilitate care were:

'It would be a good idea if some of the hospital staff came around with us to see what we have to cope with and the condition of some of the homes. We want more liaison with the hospitals.'

'If we had the facilities of the hospital, the physiotherapists etc. we could prevent a lot of these people becoming so disabled. We should go on to the ward, part of the consultant's round, and help decide when people could come out. We are the ones who have to cope with the home conditions.'

A study of the attachment of a district nurse to a surgical department showed how this could facilitate appropriately planned discharge of patients.[1] Further experiments along these lines in other situations are also needed.

Conclusions

Most of the people who die are ill or restricted for some time beforehand and need a lot of personal and nursing care. Whether this help should be given at home or in hospital will often depend on the amount of support the patient and his family can

[1] Hockey, Lisbeth, 'District nurse attached to hospital'.

be given. The district nurse was the most common professional source of such help. The descriptions given by both nurses and relatives of the ways in which the nurses helped and their relationship with other services raises doubts about:

1. The adequacy of existing district nursing services.
2. Whether district nurses are the most appropriate people to meet many current needs.
3. The effectiveness of their relationship with medical and other community services.

The demands on a service are inevitably related to its nature and extent rather than to all the needs which such a service might meet. So when the main community service is composed entirely of fully qualified and experienced nurses, demands for less skilled care may well be curtailed. Even so, 'personal care' as opposed to 'nursing care' was obviously a large part of the help given by district nurses to the people in our sample. Obviously strict demarcation lines would be inappropriate and most unhelpful in a home setting when the same patient has a wide variety of needs. It would certainly not be desirable or practical for district nurses to confine their help to skilled nursing tasks and eschew the more mundane jobs. But there is mounting evidence from other sources[1] that more effective use could be made of the skill and training of district nurses if they were backed up by less skilled people working under their supervision. This study suggests that the needs of patients and potential patients would be better served by an expansion of services to include state enrolled nurses, nursing aids and night sitters to supplement the work of the highly qualified district nurse.

[1] Hockey, Lisbeth, *Care in the Balance*, p. 115; Carstairs, Vera, *Home Nursing in Scotland*, p. 70.

7

OTHER COMMUNITY SERVICES

The help discussed in this chapter ranges from the spiritual to the material. It starts by describing the help and support given by ministers or priests, then goes on to look at some of the help which may be available through local authorities from health visitors, home helps and chiropodists. Other sorts of people who helped are then considered before describing such practical services and needs as laundry services, equipment and the additional expenditure arising from ill-health and infirmity.

The church

Apart from the district nurse the professional person who was most likely to have visited the person who died was a vicar, priest, minister or someone associated with a church. Three-tenths of the people who died had at least one visit from such a person in the year before they died.

Many received this type of help and support over some time: over half of them had more than five visits, a quarter 20 or more, but at the other end of the scale a quarter had only one or two visits. It is not possible to say how many of these visits were deliberate support of the dying and how many were regular calls to the sick, elderly or other parishioners. People living on their own were no more likely than others to have such visits, but those who were thought to have a religious faith or belief which was helpful to them[1] were more likely to be visited: 44% compared with 12% of those who were thought not to have such faith. Even more striking was the association with religious denomination: 67% of those who were Roman Catholics received such visits, 26% of those described as Church of England, 48% of other protestants and 11% of those said

[1] Question 87: 'What about ——: do you think he had a religious faith or belief which was helpful to him?'

to be atheists, agnostics or to have no religion. The proportion visited was also related to the extent and duration of their restrictions, declining from 47% of those confined to bed for three months or more to 14% of those with no restrictions. Our respondents thought that one in six of those who had not been visited would have liked a minister to call:[1] 'Yes, the vicar might have visited him. My father would have liked to talk to him I think.' The church also on occasion organised practical help, for instance the services given by the Little Sisters of the Assumption, which are described later in the chapter.

Health visitors

According to the relatives, only 8% of the people who died had been helped by a health visitor.[2] Sixty-four per cent of these had one or two visits, 21% three to five, 15% more than five. The seventy-five health visitors we saw identified eighteen persons in the sample of deaths as people they had visited.[3] Thus health visitors appeared to play a relatively small part in the care or supervision of people with a terminal illness. What did they, the district nurses and the general practitioners, feel about this? Our sample of health visitors is confined to those involved in the care of the dying or bereaved.[4] We do not know the views of other health visitors.

We asked the health visitors and district nurses we saw if they thought health visitors had a part to play in terminal home care. Ninety-five per cent of the health visitors thought so, 1%

[1] Question 54: 'Do you think he would have liked a vicar, priest or minister to visit him?'

[2] That is fifty-three people out of 703—excluding the seventy-two who had been in a hospital or institution for the twelve months before they died and ten about whom inadequate information was recorded. Of the fifty-three, thirty-two had also been helped by a district nurse, leaving 3% who had been visited by a health visitor but not a district nurse.

[3] For three of these no interview was obtained, for seven the data from the relatives tallied with that from the health visitors, for the other eight there was some discrepancy—the relative apparently forgot in two, was unaware of it for one, described the health visitor as a welfare visitor (one), the health visitor identified the wrong person (one), and recorded help which did not amount to a visit (three).

[4] Just over a third of those we saw had been involved only in the care of bereaved and not with any dying patients. They were not asked the questions about the care of the terminally ill.

thought not, the others gave qualified answers. But this finding is not surprising in view of the nature of our sample. It would be interesting to know the opinions of health visitors not working in this field.

The district nurses were more divided: 55% thought health visitors had a part to play, 43% thought not, 2% were uncertain. The two main points of view are illustrated by these quotations:

> 'They are another visitor going in and reassuring them. They can offer services that perhaps have not been thought of by the nurse. You can often work together instead of the nurse being on her own, especially in a big case.'

> 'They don't do anything—just pass it on to us anyway. They never roll up their sleeves and do anything.'

General practitioners were asked a different question: whether they found the health visitor services very helpful, moderately helpful or not helpful for patients at home with terminal illness. Twenty-eight per cent said they were very helpful, 25% moderately, 47% not helpful. (This was in contrast to their reaction to the district nursing service which 85% found 'very helpful' and 15% 'moderately helpful'.) Again, general practitioners with a health visitor attached to the practice were more appreciative of their usefulness: 48% of those doctors and 12% of the others thought health visitors very helpful and the proportions describing them as not helpful were 25% of doctors with an attachment and 62% of the others.

General practitioners usually instigated district nursing care; 91% of the relatives and 85% of the nurses said they had done so for the people in our sample. They were also the people who had most often arranged for a health visitor to call, but they made such arrangements much less often, both relatively and absolutely, for about three-fifths of the people visited by a health visitor, that is for about 5% of all the people who died. If health visitors are to play an effective part in this type of care under the present system, clearly general practitioners need to be more convinced of their usefulness.

The type of help health visitors give is less direct than that given by district nurses and therefore possibly less easily recognised and appreciated. Only 9% of the relatives who said the deceased had been visited by a health visitor said she had helped with either personal or nursing care. And the health visitors themselves described the help they gave to the people in our sample mainly as 'supervision only'. This implies that their liaison with other services needs to be effective. They were more critical than district nurses of the inadequacies of other services. Thirty-two per cent of the health visitors, compared with 22% of district nurses, regarded the home help service as 'very inadequate', and 56% of the health visitors, 82% of the district nurses, thought the district nursing service in their area was adequate. At the same time the health visitors were also more likely to think that relatives sought admission to hospital rather than accepting responsibility for home care: 20% of them thought this, 9% of district nurses.

Health visitors, more often than either district nurses or general practitioners, thought that unsuitable housing, inadequate home nursing services and inadequate supporting

TABLE 49 *Views of health visitors, district nurses and general practitioners on what prevents more people being looked after in the community rather than in hospital*

	Health visitors	*District nurses*	*General practitioners*
	%	%	%
Unsuitable housing	81	58	60
Unwillingness of relatives to look after them	92	85	90
Absence of suitable relatives	92	94	93
Inadequate home nursing service	39	21	25
Inadequate supporting services	71	42	33
Tendency of hospital doctors to admit unnecessarily	5	7	5
Tendency not to discharge people when reasonable	11	16	7
Overwork of general practitioner	29	28	27
None of these	3	—	—
Number of professionals (=100%)	75	507	283

services played a part in preventing more people being looked after in the community (see Table 49). Presumably the social orientation of their training made them more aware of these considerations.

The home help service was mentioned most often as an example of inadequate supporting services. One health visitor was particularly vehement about this:

> 'There isn't sufficient home help to cover the old people. It's cut down to a minimum. The old people are being cut back not the flaming schools. There isn't sufficient money allocated to the old people. It's very wrong to cut down on the home help service to the old people.'

Home helps

Ten per cent of the people who died had been helped by a home help during the last twelve months of their lives.[1] Relatives of another 13% thought they could have done with some help from one,[2] and they felt 44% of those who did have some help could have done with it more often. On these two counts it would seem to be the most inadequate of the community services we asked about. Only a quarter of the general practitioners regarded the home help service in their area as 'adequate', just over a quarter thought it 'very inadequate'. Some comments were:

> 'It's inadequate in time only. As a general rule they are a dedicated band of very hard working people, some of whom will do jobs and work hours well beyond their normal call of duty' (rather inadequate).

> 'There should be a far greater number of home helps. The shortage is due to lack of finance. In fact there is a waiting list here of people who want to be a home help but the

[1] Those who had been in a hospital or institution for a year or more before they died have been excluded from this section.

[2] Hunt, Audrey, in *The Home Help Service in England and Wales*, p. 24, reported: 'There are probably at least as many households in need of home help among the elderly population as are currently receiving it', and: 'There are possibly twice as many households with a chronic sick housewife in need of home help as are currently receiving it.'

County won't pay. It's a disgrace I think' (very inadequate).

'Home helps can only give each case one or two hours a week. It's not enough to keep a helpless patient out of hospital. I have a case in mind where adequate home help would make all the difference. I have a patient with carcinomatosis. She has had an arm amputated and is really very ill. She discharged herself from hospital because they can really do nothing for her. Her sister, a full-time ward sister in a London hospital, gives up her weekends to caring for her. Another sister, with a family of her own living six miles away, goes in each day and sometimes has to sleep in. A daily home help would be the best answer in this case. The district nurses go in but they haven't time to see to things in the house—or meals' (very inadequate).

'Many more people who should have a home help do not do so because of the charges involved' (adequate).

'Sometimes old people are left without one for some days. At best their services are rather infrequent' (rather inadequate).

Altogether a third of the general practitioners thought that inadequate supporting services—other than home nursing—prevented more people being looked after in the community rather than in hospital.

Nearly all the home helps did cleaning, about a third helped with cooking, a third with shopping and just over a quarter with washing clothes. About one in ten did things other than housework and shopping. Half the people with a home help had her once a week or less often, just over a third had her more than once a week but not as often as daily, one in eight had her daily. Just over half, 57%, had help for over a year: few, 8%, had it for less than a month. One of the complaints made by general practitioners was about the difficulty of organising short-term help quickly:

'Say you have a patient with an acute illness—you telephone for a home help—someone then has to come to assess the situation and then you might get someone a week later—

the need has gone. It's impossible to get immediate help when the need is greatest' (very inadequate).

Chiropody

Eleven per cent of the people who died were said to have been helped by a chiropodist in the year before they died. This is fewer than might be expected from the results of another study which focused entirely on foot problems and found that 29% of the people aged 65 and over, and 14% of those aged 45–64 reported some professional treatment for their feet during a six-month period.[1] These findings suggest that relatives under-reported this type of care, probably forgetting about it when confronted with the other problems of terminal illness. Nearly all those who said their relative had been helped by a chiropodist mentioned this when we asked if the person had needed help with cutting toenails. Nearly half, 48%, of the people who died had needed help with this and a fifth of them (a tenth of the total sample) had this done, at any rate sometimes, by a chiropodist. Husbands or wives helped a third of them, daughters a quarter, other relatives just over a quarter and district nurses a sixth. Relatives thought another 7% could have done with some help from a chiropodist. Middle-class people were more likely to have had help from a chiropodist than working-class people: 15% compared with 8%. Similar class differences were found on the other study.[1]

Other helpers

Twelve per cent of the people who died were said to have been helped by people from other organisations.[2] These included welfare officers from their work, people from the hospital, officials from the Department of Health and Social Security, people from the Salvation Army, the associations for the physically handicapped and for the general welfare of the blind.

[1] Clarke, May, *Trouble with Feet*, p. 42.

[2] Question 52: 'Can I check the various sorts of official people who helped —— during the last 12 months of his life (while he was at home)? During that time did he have any help from or was he ever visited by a district nurse, health visitor, other nurse, home help, special laundry service, chiropodist, vicar, priest or minister, any other official or voluntary service (SPECIFY)?'

Most of these had come just once or twice to find out whether people were getting the help they needed. Others who helped more directly were night sitters from the 'Marie Curie' or the 'Cancer fund' and the Little Sisters of the Assumption. The last service aims to concentrate on the type of help other people do not or cannot provide, and to give complete care to families, caring for children when the mother is ill, and helping the father to stay at work. They give night care, nursing care, help with cleaning, look after children, prepare meals, shop, lend equipment and liaise with other services. As well as people with terminal illness they help those who are chronically ill, those with mental illness, the subnormal and problem families. They had a centre in one of our study areas. Some of the Sisters there were trained nurses, another a social worker and two were trained in household management. Others collected money. Most of the people they helped had been referred by general practitioners. Several of the district nurses in that area told us about the service: 'they will do anything at all'; 'they can go in and give a twenty-four hour service'; 'they will go to anyone not only R.C.s'. But only two people in our sample seemed to have been helped by them. One was a woman in her early sixties who lived with her husband and had died at home from cancer. The nuns had come in six times a day to do dressings and stayed until eleven o'clock at night. 'They'd have stayed all night if we'd asked. They were just angels. You can't describe how you feel. They'd make you laugh too.' Obviously a small organisation can give such intensive help only to a few people.

Laundry for the incontinent

Over a quarter of the people who died had at some stage soiled their bed linen while they were at home. The ways in which people coped with this are shown in Table 50. Several had used more than one method.

Washing at home and disposable pads or sheets were the most common ways of coping. Even when people had a washing machine they sometimes found this a distressing and tiring chore.

Coping with laundry sometimes tipped the balance between home and hospital care. A daughter whose mother had been

TABLE 50 *Coping with soiled bed linen*

	%
Special laundry service	5
Ordinary laundry service	7
Launderette	7
Washed at home by hand	29
Washed at home by machine	41
Disposable pads	37
Disposable sheets	17
Others[a]	22
Number with soiled bed linen to cope with at home in last year of person's life (=100%)	198

[a] Others includes colostomy bags, cotton wool, sanitary pads and 'bits of sheet'.

ill for many years said that when her mother became incontinent in the last week of her life: 'I couldn't cope. She was getting through nighties like wildfire. That's why I rang the doctor. I didn't think she was as bad as she was; it was just that I couldn't cope.' Her mother died of heart failure and bronchitis within twenty-four hours of being admitted to hospital.

One in six of those who did not have a special laundry service would have liked one.

A laundry service needs to be frequent and efficient to deal with the needs of the incontinent. Using disposable pads or sheets may seem more appropriate, but presents other difficul-

TABLE 51 *Disposing of disposables*

	%
Burning indoors in fireplace	26
Burning indoors in stove	10
Burning outdoors on open fire	21
Burning outdoors in incinerator	26
Dustbin	20
Special collection	—
Other	6
Number using disposables (=100%)[a]	96

[a] Excluding those who had been in a hospital or institution for a year or more before they died.

ties. Ways in which people got rid of disposables are shown in Table 51.

No one had disposables collected by a special collection, and the relatives of a fifth of those using disposables said getting rid of them had presented a problem.

Equipment

A washing machine, spin dryer, car and telphone may make it easier to look after people who are old or sick at home. Table 52 shows the proportions of households in which the dead person had lived which had these and the proportions in which the respondents thought it might have been helpful to have had them.

TABLE 52 *Household equipment*

	Proportion of dead person's household with equipment	*Proportion in which it would have been helpful based on those without it*[a]
	%	
Washing machine	56	32% (253)
Spin dryer	44	37% (325)
Car	36	26% (374)
Telephone	35	51% (382)
None of these	31	—
Number of households[b]	604	—

[a] Figures in brackets are the numbers on which the percentages are based (=100%).
[b] Excludes those in hospital or institution for a year or more before they died and those under 65 who died unexpectedly without any previous restrictions.

Half those without a telephone thought it would have been useful.

> 'We have quite a long way to go for one and then it's not always in order and if someone was ill and it was night time I wouldn't go down those streets—not safe.'

> 'We had it in the other house—couldn't afford it here. I think you should have it with a blind man.'

> 'A telephone the night she died would have been helpful' (died of heart attack aged 65).

> 'A telephone would have been a godsend instead of her having to use the call box.'

But not everyone is used to telephoning, and if they had a telephone they would need some help before they could use it:

> 'It would have been useful but I've never used a telephone in my life. I suppose there are ways of learning. The neighbours used to phone for me or I went up to the clinic' (wife of 76 whose husband died of cancer).

This last woman did not think a washing machine or spin dryer would have been useful although her husband had loss of bladder control for over a year before he died, and was only in hospital for the last four days of his life.

> 'I've seen such things. My husband's wages were very small. We only got £2 a week when I first came here. He only used to get £5 at the end. The rent was 10/- a week.'

And a daughter whose father had had Parkinson's disease, arteriosclerosis and double incontinence said about a washing machine:

> 'Mother wouldn't use one. She hated any electric appliance. I begged her to let me buy a washing machine but she wouldn't. She did everything the hard way.'

A fifth of the respondents said there were other pieces of equipment the person who died would have found helpful. Some of the things they would have liked were:

> 'A gadget for picking up things from the floor. I didn't know there was such a thing until recently.'

> 'A cage for her feet. We used a fireguard as makeshift. She had awful bunions, the weight of the bedclothes was too much.'

> 'Something to keep his legs and feet warm. It was an

awful problem to keep him warm with the cradle holding the blanket.'

A quarter of the people who died or our respondents had spent money on equipment. The proportions needing different sorts of equipment are shown in Table 53.[1]

TABLE 53 *Proportion needing various items of equipment*

	%
Backrest	17
Hoist	2
Special bed	3
Wheelchair	10
Crutches/stick/walking aid	18
Commode	30
Hearing aid	7
Bedpan or bottle	28
Mackintosh sheet	26
Pads to protect bed	17
Extra linen	11
Other	13
None[a]	39
Number of deaths excluding those in hospital or institution for whole year (=100%)	697

[a] This question was not asked for unexpected deaths of people under 65. These have been included as not needing any equipment.

A fifth of those who were thought to need a wheelchair, and one in eight of those needing a hearing aid, did not have one. Most of the wheelchairs and hearing aids were obtained through official or voluntary sources, but a substantial proportion had been bought by the deceased or their families. This can be seen from Table 54. Most people either had or bought any extra linen needed, but official and voluntary sources met about a third of such needs.

[1] Question 44: 'Did —— need any equipment like: [things listed in Table 53] or anything else?'

TABLE 54 *Acquisition of needed equipment*

	Back rest, hoist, other furniture	*Wheelchair*	*Crutches, stick, walking aid*	*Commode*	*Hearing aid*	*Bedpan or bottle*	*Mackintosh sheet, extra linen*
How acquired	%	%	%	%	%	%	%
Bought	23	14	19	23	25	35	27
Borrowed, given, supplied or hired from:							
Relatives	3	—	3	4	—	2	4
Friends/neighbours	6	3	4	13	—	6	3
Official or voluntary sources	39	60	36	20	54	34	35
Already had them	9	2	37	33	8	17	25
Not acquired	20	21	1	7	13	6	6
Number needing equipment (=100%)	223[a]	67	122	205	48	184	276[a]

[a] For these, which can include more than one item of equipment for the same person, the base is the number of different sources or items.

Financial help

The items on which people had additional expenditure during the last twelve months are shown in Table 55.[1] Heating, fares or petrol, equipment and special foods were the most frequent additional costs.

Over a third of the respondents thought that when people in the dead person's household had been faced with additional expenditure it had not been easy for them to find the extra money.[2]

A husband whose wife aged 62 died of mitral stenosis, having

[1] Question 48: 'Did you and/or he have any additional expenditure during the last 12 months of his life because of his illness/disability/old age on such things as: heating, laundry, special food, extra help, prescription charges, other medicines, fares or petrol, equipment or anything else?'

[2] Question 48a: 'Would you say it was quite easy for you/him to find that extra money or not?'

TABLE 55 *Proportion with additional expenditure on different items*[a]

	%
Heating	37
Laundry	19
Special food	22
Extra help	10
Prescription charges	16
Other medicines	11
Fares, petrol	35
Equipment	25
Other	9
None[b]	34
Number excluding those in hospital or institution all year (=100%)	668

[a] Includes expenditure by the dead person and the respondent if the respondent was in the same household as the dead person.

[b] This question was not asked about those who died unexpectedly with no restrictions. They have been included as having no additional expenditure.

been ill for two and a half years, had additional expenditure on prescription charges and fares:

> 'We spent a lot of money—she needed more and more pills to keep her going. When I asked about the cost of the tablets the chemist said she wasn't old enough to get any refund. She was going to hospital about once a fortnight at the end. This was expensive [the return fare was over five shillings]. My daughter used to pay her mother's fare.'

A wife whose husband died of cancer said: 'the prescriptions were a strain until a friend told me about being able to get them free for permanent illness. I asked my doctor about this and he gave me the special form.'

Additional expenditure was related to the length and type of restriction. This is shown in Table 56. Prescription charges were the exception to this, partly because they do not apply to people aged 65 or more. They were mentioned in connection with only 4% of the deaths of people of that age compared with 41% of the deaths of people under 65. People with certain types of chronic illness could also claim exemption from these charges; but over a fifth of those who had been severely restricted or confined to bed for three months or more still reported this as an additional expense, and this proportion was over half among such deaths of people under 65.

A wife whose husband died of cancer had additional expenditure on heating, laundry, special food, prescription

TABLE 56 *Additional expenditure for people with different types of restrictions*

	Bedridden for three months or longer	*Confined mainly to bed for three months or longer*	*Severely restricted for three months or longer*	*Moderately restricted for three months or longer*	*Other restriction for three months or longer*	*Restricted for less than three months*	*No restrictions*
Additional expenditure on:	%	%	%	%	%	%	%
Heating	67	54	47	38	28	32	12
Laundry	37	27	24	19	11	15	6
Special food	42	34	26	21	18	16	9
Extra help	17	11	16	10	11	3	6
Prescription charges	14	24	21	12	16	21	7
Other medicines	20	18	13	8	10	9	6
Fares, petrol	48	41	42	35	29	38	12
Equipment	47	43	29	24	22	17	5
Other	12	12	10	9	9	10	4
None[a]	17	11	18	28	38	39	75
Extra money easy to find:	%	%	%	%	%	%	%
Yes	52	42	51	46	48	41	15
No	31	47	31	26	14	20	10
None needed[a]	17	11	18	28	38	39	75
Number, excluding those in hospital or institution all year (=100%)[b]	65	74	108	103	104	120	121

[a] This question was not asked about those who died unexpectedly with no previous restrictions. They have been included as having no additional expenditure.

[b] Those for whom inadequate information was obtained have been excluded when calculating percentages,

charges, other medicines (Veganin) and fares and said it had not been easy to find the extra money. She had not asked anyone for help as 'I don't suppose anyone would give it to me' (husband a garage manager).

> 'It wasn't easy it was a lot of expense but we didn't have to ask for help. You don't reckon things like that when your husband's ill, you get what he needs. Prescription charges were 7/6*d*. a week, sometimes 10/-—stacks and stacks of tablets went away that weren't suitable for him. And heating—he was so cold all the time we had to have extra electric fires and blankets'—also additional expenditure on special food and fares (husband a butcher).

A daughter whose mother died at 78 of heart failure but had been severely restricted for over a year by breathlessness said her mother had additional expense on heating and did not find it easy. They had asked the 'Social Security man but he said he couldn't help. He never did one solitary thing for us—we're not pushers, mind, if we'd pushed maybe we'd have got something, but he never once helped Mam.'

Earlier in Chapter 2 we saw that just over a fifth of the people who died were said to have needed financial help. One in seven of those reported to need it did not get help from anyone. The source of help most frequently mentioned, for three-fifths of those in need, was Social Security. But it is likely that our data about this were incomplete. Financial help was the one type of care more often given by sons (16%), than by daughters (11%).

Conclusions

Community services for the old and ill are haphazard in their distribution and generally inadequate. This is particularly true for the home help service. But its inadequacies have been well documented.[1] Research is no panacea in itself. People, and particularly local authorities and central government, have to be persuaded to take action. This generally involves spending more money. It is not enough to rely on the dedication and self-

[1] Hunt, Audrey, op. cit.; Harris, Amelia I., *Social Welfare for the Elderly*, Vol. 1, p. 66.

sacrifice of the individuals already working in the service. People who can tolerate over-work and low wages are likely to be idealists but a few may also be martyrs and masochists. Those needed to support the elderly and dying need self-confidence and sympathy. They should be supported by appropriate recognition, in terms of both money and status, of the value of the job they are doing.

One service for which the community does not often accept responsibility at the moment is the provision of telephones for elderly people who live alone. A recent experimental study in Hull among people who were housebound suggested that there was a strong case for such a service in terms of its potential use in emergencies but that it would also add to the social contacts and general convenience of the people.[1]

Even when services exist other studies have shown that people often do not know about them or use them.[2] This may be the reason why so many of the chronically-ill who were under 65 were paying prescription charges, though probably only some of them would have been exempt.

Voluntary organisations may attempt to fill some of the gaps in our statutory services, but it is clear that many of these gaps ought not to exist. Voluntary workers should be able to fill their traditional role of meeting needs as yet unrecognised or unaccepted as community responsibilities. The needs of people who are dying at home, for personal, nursing and other types of care should surely be met by statutory community services when they cannot be met by their own relatives and friends. These people should not have to rely on the inevitably haphazard charity of voluntary associations. In practice the alternatives were often to do without or to be helped by relatives and friends.

[1] Gregory, Peter and Young, Michael, *Lifeline Telephone Service for the Elderly*.

[2] Lance, Hilary, 'Transport services in general practice'; Meyrick, R. L., 'A geriatric survey in general practice'; Meyrick, R. L. and Cox, A., 'A geriatric survey repeated'.

8

CARE FROM RELATIVES AND FRIENDS

In the last four chapters we have considered the care given by health and welfare services and voluntary organisations to people during the last year of their lives. But earlier, in Chapter 2, we saw that relatives were the most common source of help during this time. In this chapter we describe the relatives and friends who helped and what they did for the people who died and then discuss the implications for both the helpers and the helped.

The helpers and the helped[1]

On average people who died had been helped by three relatives and friends,[2] and this did not vary with the marital status of the people who died. But the sorts of people who helped were naturally very different, as can be seen from Table 57. For married people three-fifths of their helpers were members of their nuclear family—husband, wife, sons and daughters. People who were widowed were as likely as those who were married to be helped by a son but they had more assistance from daughters. The widowed were more dependent than the married on other relatives such as grand-children, nieces and nephews, and cousins and on friends and neighbours, but the single, with no immediate family to help them (except that 3% of their helpers were parents), relied most heavily on their neighbours, friends and more distant relatives.

[1] People who had been in a hospital or institution for a year or more before they died and those who died unexpectedly before they were 65 have not been included in this section.

[2] Question 49: 'Can I check that I've got a note of all the different friends and relations who helped —— in any of the ways shown on the card?' CHECK Respondent, others in the same household, other relatives, other friends or neighbours. The card listed all the different types of help described in Chapter 2.

TABLE 57 *Helpers and marital status of the person who died*

	Single	*Married*	*Widowed, divorced, separated*	*All*
	%	%	%	%
Wife	—	20	1[a]	11
Husband	—	10	1[a]	6
Daughter	—	17	27	19
Son	—	14	13	12
Daughter- or son-in-law	—	6	16	9
Sister or brother	24	4	5	7
Sister- or brother-in-law	8	4	1	3
Other relative	23	7	14	11
Friend, neighbour or other person	45	18	22	22
Number of helpers (=100%)	194	936	658	1,817
Average number of people who helped[b]	2·8	2·7	2·8	2·7

[a] In these instances the husband or wife who had helped died before the spouse they were helping.

[b] Those who were in a hospital or institution for a year or more before they died and those who died unexpectedly before they were 65 have been excluded.

Ties with brothers and sisters seemed strongest for the single. Nearly a quarter of their helpers were brothers and sisters, compared with one in twenty-five of those helping the married or widowed. Thirty-six per cent of the people who died had no brothers or sisters living in England or Wales, and this proportion was similar for the married, single and widowed. But whereas 77% of the single had seen all their brothers and sisters who lived in England and Wales during the year before their death rather less, 62%, of the married and widowed had done so.[1]

The married and widowed depended more on their children: 84% of them had children living in England and Wales and 93% of those had seen all their children in the last year of their

[1] This difference might have occurred by chance ($p < 0 \cdot 10$) but taken with the other findings it seems suggestive.

lives. More daughters helped than sons but similar numbers of sons-in-law and daughters-in-law were involved in care and more sons (0·13 on average) than daughters-in-law (0·03). So sons do not seem just to delegate the care of their parents to their wives; but, whereas people had help from an average of 0·67 daughters and daughters' husbands the comparable number for sons and sons' wives was 0·45.

With the strength of these family ties and the large part played by wives, husbands, daughters and sons in looking after the people who died it may seem surprising that single people had nearly as many helpers as the married and widowed. Part of the reason for this was their greater reliance on brothers and sisters and on more distant relatives such as nieces and cousins. But they had more help from friends and neighbours. For them ties of friendship and neighbourliness seem to compensate for their lack of immediate family.

TABLE 58 *Helpers and household composition of the person who died*

	On own	*With spouse only*	*With relatives of same or older generation*	*With relatives of a younger generation*	*With unrelated people only, in guesthouse etc.*
	%	%	%	%	%
Wife	—	21	4	9	—
Husband	1[a]	13	2	3	—
Daughter	23	16	3	23	—
Son	10	9	3	16	2
Daughter- or son-in-law	11	7	2	12	—
Sister or brother	4	2	34	5	—
Sister- or brother-in-law	3	3	7	3	2
Other relative	15	7	13	14	8
Friends, neighbours or other person	33	22	32	15	88
Number of helpers (=100%)	232	490	139	906	50
Average number of people who helped	2·5	2·3	2·6	3·2	1·8

[a] This man died before the wife he had been helping.

People living alone relied on friends and neighbours rather less than single people, partly because many of them had help from daughters and sons. This can be seen from Table 58, which also shows that those least likely to have help from unrelated people were those living with relatives of a younger generation.

Those living with just their spouse or with unrelated people or in a guesthouse had fewest helpers. The average of 1·8 for this last group has been inflated by one woman who lived in a convent where all the sisters took turns to look after her. Among the others the average was 1·4.

There were only three people in the sample who had no helpers or contact with close relatives in the last year of their lives:

> A single man of 65 died from heart trouble after being in hospital five weeks. Previously he had lived with his landlord and the landlord's deaf and dumb son. The landlord said he had not needed any help while he was at home but described his health as 'No good. He drank too much. Beer was his trouble.' He had a brother and sister who lived within half an hour's journey but had not seen them at all in the year before he died.

> A man of 69 lived on his own. He was separated from his wife and the friend we interviewed said 'No one knows where [she lives]. They advertised. He never talked about her—never mentioned her.' The friends who had known him for over five years did not know if he had any children or brothers or sisters, although 'He used to come every Saturday for a cup of tea and a smoke'. He died accidentally from a fall off a ladder.

> The third, also a man of about 68, lived in a bedsitting room and looked after himself. We interviewed his landlady who said 'We didn't know anything about him. He was a man of few words. You couldn't have a conversation with him. He had his own room and looked after himself. Every two weeks the rooms were cleaned and the bed linen changed. We didn't know anything about his history at all and we didn't probe. These people who live

in bedsitters and look after themselves like to be left alone. They don't want to be fussed around.' He had lived there for less than a year having moved from other digs where he had full board. He had a number of sisters who lived within two hours' journey but the only time they visited 'was to take his things after he died'. He died in hospital of broncho-pneumonia but also had cancer.

Those living alone and those living with people unrelated to them were less likely to have children or siblings living in England and Wales than others. The proportions without children were 41% of those living alone, 95% of those living with unrelated people, 19% of the others, and the proportions with no siblings 49%, 63% and 32% respectively. Twenty-three per cent of those living alone, 32% of those with unrelated people, and 6% of the others had neither children nor siblings living in England and Wales. Presumably this was one of the reasons why they did not live with relatives.

Up to now we have looked at variations in the numbers and relationships of the people who helped with the marital status and household composition of the person who died. Age, sex and social class made little difference to the number of helpers. But a more important question is, how did the numbers and relationships vary with their needs? Table 59 shows how the number of people who helped varied with the number of symptoms reported for the person who died, the extent of their restriction and the number of different ways in which they needed help.

The more things there are to be done, the more people in the informal network of relatives and friends are involved in helping. But, as we discussed earlier, this apparent matching of needs and care may be something of an illusion. If relatives are around they may help with things the person would otherwise have managed to do for himself.

What is perhaps more revealing is that the number of helpers did not appear to increase with the length of time the person needed help: there was no association between the number of helpers and the period over which the help was needed. Those who were able and willing to help seemed to do so when the need was recognised, but they did not recruit further helpers

TABLE 59 *Average number of relatives and friends helping in different situations*

Number of symptoms reported			*Restriction*		
None or one	1·5	(67)	Bedridden or mainly confined to bed for three months or longer	3·4	(136)
Two	1·8	(76)	Severely restricted for three months or longer	3·0	(107)
Three	2·5	(77)	Other restriction for three months or longer	2·6	(204)
Four	2·7	(94)	Any restriction for less than three months	2·8	(111)
Five	2·9	(86)	None	1·3	(70)
Six	3·2	(73)			
Seven	3·2	(61)			
Eight or more	3·8	(112)			
Number of things needed help with[a]					
None	0·2	(64)			
1–4	1·9	(107)			
5–9	2·8	(155)			
10–14	3·2	(159)			
15–19	3·8	(129)			
20+	4·1	(31)			

The figures in brackets are the denominators on which the averages are based.

[a] That is, the things we asked specifically about, but relatives and friends helping in other ways have also been included.

when the same need persisted over a long time, only when additional needs were perceived.

This is in contrast to the findings in Chapter 6 which showed that the district nurse more often helped when the person needed short-term rather than long-term care. So people with long-term needs who stayed at home were particularly dependent on their relatives and friends. How often did the relatives and friends help and what did they do?

The frequency and nature of help

Most of the helpers who lived in the same household as the person who died helped every day:[1] 87% did so, 93% of the women helpers, 77% of the men.

Inevitably, the help given by those not living in the same household was less frequent. Even so, three-tenths of them

[1] Question 49: 'Did they help regularly or occasionally?' IF REGULARLY 'How often?'

helped every day; over a third of the daughters and daughters-in-law living outside who helped did so, as did over one in five of the sons and sons-in-law. Nearly a third of the friends and neighbours who helped did this daily.

Most of the people outside the household who helped (four-fifths) lived within half an hour's journey of the person who died. This proportion was naturally higher, 95%, for friends and neighbours than for relatives, 72%. Sons and daughters tended to travel further than sons-in-law and daughters-in-law to help, and brothers and sisters had relatively the longest journeys. This is shown in Table 60.

TABLE 60 *Length of journey for helpers outside the household*

	Son	*Daughter*	*Son-in-law*	*Daughter-in-law*	*Brother or sister*	*Other relative*	*Friend, neighbour or others*	*All helpers outside household*
	%	%	%	%	%	%	%	%
Within 10 minutes' walk	23	31	33	38	19	32	82	47
Within half-hour journey	47	40	50	54	45	36	13	33
Half an hour but less than 1 hour	13	14	5	2	15	15	3	10
An hour but less than 2 hours	8	7	2	4	10	10	1	5
Two hours or more	9	8	10	2	11	7	1	5
Number of helpers outside household (=100%)	121	188	40	55	67	188	336	995

The sorts of things different people did are shown in Table 61. Daughters were not only more likely than sons to have helped at all, but when they did so they also helped with more things. Friends and neighbours rarely undertook nursing care; the way they most often helped was by doing some housework, but a third of them helped with self care and a fifth had sometimes sat with the person at night.

TABLE 61 *Nature of help given by different people*

	Wife or husband	*Daughters*	*Sons*	*Other relatives*	*Friends neighbours or other people*
	%	%	%	%	%
Self care	80	62	44	47	33
Nursing	61	39	14	18	9
Night	55	34	31	24	21
Social	61	52	39	33	26
Financial	[a]	6	15	3	—
Housework	22[b]	50[b]	21	35	44
Number of helpers (=100%)	289	341	218	553	411
Average number of different things helped with[c]	8·0	6·3	3·8	3·8	2·9

[a] Married couples were not regarded as helping each other financially.
[b] When the person normally did the housework they were not regarded as helping the person who died with this.
[c] Of all things listed in Table 16.

In general, those living in the same household were more likely to help in nearly all the different ways listed. They had helped with an average of nearly seven things compared with just over three for those not living in the same household.

Some idea of the intensity of the care that people outside the household gave, and the length of time over which they gave it, is suggested by the number of times they saw the person who died during the last year of their lives. A third of the daughters who helped had seen the person 300 times or more, and a further 56% had seen them on fifty or more occasions, 11% less often. Comparable proportions for sons were 24% seeing them 300 times or more, 60% between fifty and 300, 16% less often. Sons-in-law had seen them about as often as sons, but daughters-in-law rather less often than daughters. Of the friends, neighbours and other unrelated people who helped, a fifth had seen them at least 300 times in the year, half on 50–300 occasions, another one in seven twenty times or more and one in eight less frequently. So most of the people who helped had many contacts with the person who died and helped in a number of ways.

What of the people who are part of these statistics? These examples illustrate some of the different but more common situations.

A man of 89 had received almost all the help he needed from his wife whom we interviewed. She was over 80 herself. He was said to have been moderately restricted for over six months. 'He had an operation for a prostate gland three years ago and he got worse.' Among other things he had needed help getting into and out of the bath for over six months; and his wife said that for over a year she had needed, but not got, help with cleaning the house and washing clothes. In the last few days he had also needed help to get in and out of bed, to go to the lavatory and he had needed someone to sit with him at night. Eventually he was taken into hospital, where he died, after less than twenty-four hours, of pneumonia. 'I wish I hadn't let him go, but I couldn't cope, I was so tired myself.' The only help the wife said she received was 'with the rent from the National Assistance'. The husband's brother and sister lived quite near and visited a few times in the last year, 'but are old themselves'.

By contrast, another couple in their late sixties received help from many sources. The wife was said to have been a little restricted for over six months, and needed help with washing herself, getting to the lavatory, drinks at night, shopping, cooking and housework for over three months. The husband (our respondent) was the main source of help, but a district nurse, a sister-in-law, a home help, nieces and various friends also helped regularly. For example, apart from the husband, four people were said to have helped at night. The husband had a list of twenty-two friends who had all helped with shopping, cleaning, washing and cooking, which he had sent to his daughter-in-law so that she could write a personal letter of thanks.

A single woman aged 81 had had heart trouble for over five years and slowly deteriorated during that time. For the last year of her life she was unable to leave the house. She lived with her sister (our respondent) who was also single and in her late seventies, who gave her nearly all of the many kinds of personal help she needed and who looked after all the cooking, shopping, etc. that was necessary. The only other people who helped were a home help who did the cleaning and a neighbour who did the shopping when our respondent broke her wrist. Looking after her sister meant that she was 'more tied to the house certainly, though that didn't trouble me—but after she took to bed [over three months before she died] I only went out when I had to'. The experience had also made her reflect about what the future held for her, now she was living alone. 'I don't want to give up my home—in a way I'd like someone—but I'm afraid to—you might get someone and not be happy. I do wonder who'll look after me when I need it though? I used to say that to her.'

A widow aged 81 lived with her unmarried daughter (our respondent). 'She had poor near vision, she was developing cataracts—so she was likely to fall. Her legs were uncertain.' The daughter was the only source of help for the many kinds of self care which were needed such as getting in and out of the bath, dressing and getting to the lavatory. The daughter also read to her and wrote letters for her. A nephew, brother-in-law or friend occasionally took the mother out, and occasionally a neighbour helped with the shopping. She needed help at night with a bedpan, and the daughter slept in the same room. 'I asked for night nurses but nobody knew of any. I went to our doctor saying as I was getting up every night two or three times was there any help I could have. He said he didn't think so, but would get the geriatric doctor from St A's to come to see her. He said what a beautiful house we had and told my mother how lucky she was to be in such pleasant surroundings. I said this didn't help me—so he said he would have her in for a fortnight later in the year so that I could get away.' She eventually entered the hospital less than a week before she died of a chest infection plus anaemia and cardiac trouble. When she went into hospital the daughter was 'distressed for her in a way, but relieved that I could have some rest at night'.

An 84-year-old widow, living on her own, was said to have been moderately restricted for more than a year. 'She was getting on and needed a bit of help with the shopping, cooking her dinner and keeping the home tidy.' Our respondent, a neighbour, came in daily and provided all the help she needed. 'I was glad to do little things for her. If I made a cake, I would make one for her as well. It is sad to be old and living on your own. I liked helping the old lady.' The only other person said to have helped was another neighbour—'she helped a lot at first, then her husband was taken ill and she could not help much'. The widow died of a heart attack in our respondent's arms. Her only near relative was a nephew, but he did not come to see her in the year before she died.

Visiting at home and hospital

In describing the help given by relatives and friends we have not counted just visiting someone, whether at home or in hospital, as helping. But such contacts with relatives and friends probably meant a good deal to those who died.

On average people were visited at home but not helped by between two and three close relatives (children, brothers or sisters or others) in the year before they died.

All but 4% of the people who had been in hospital at any time during the year before they died had been visited by relatives or friends while they were there. Most of the few who had not had been admitted very shortly before their death; the others had been in for a year or more.

Nearly nine-tenths had three or more different visitors. Some idea of the amount of visiting done by friends and relatives is given by the fact that nearly a quarter of the people who had been in hospital at all during the year before they died had been visited at least fifty times in that year by the person we interviewed and another quarter had been visited on twenty to fifty occasions.

More respondents, 87%, thought the visiting arrangements satisfactory, only 6% felt them unsatisfactory and 7% had reservations. Most of the few critical comments were about their problems in fitting visits in with their work, home and travel arrangements:

A woman whose 46-year-old husband had been in hospital for six weeks before he died of cancer described how she used to leave home at 7.15 a.m. to get to work, then she had to do the shopping at 5.30 p.m., catch the six o'clock bus to get to the hospital, and eventually got home at nine o'clock. 'Three hours for a one hour visit.'

> 'I would have preferred to visit at any time because as it was I had to rush to the hospital straight from work to get there in time and never seemed to be able to relax after the rushing about.' (A son who had visited his widowed mother over fifty times while she was in hospital. The journey took between one and two hours.)

> A man who visited his wife every day explained: 'I could only go in the evenings and had to get someone to look after our little girl. I work for myself so in a way it was easier but it was my money I was losing when I had work to do.'

Others just wanted more opportunity to be with the person who was dying:

> 'I felt I should have been able to see her more often. They must have known what was wrong and that she hadn't long to live' (husband whose wife died of leukaemia after being in hospital for less than a week).

But those who said the arrangements were satisfactory were not all without problems.

One daughter whose mother had been in an old people's home for ten years used to have to spend the weekend with her mother's sister aged 89 in order to visit her mother. 'If you don't have a car it's a terrible place to get to. The only thing I have against these homes—there's nowhere you can talk privately. All the other old people are listening because they've nothing else to do poor old things.'

> 'It was difficult with the children. I felt he might die any time and certainly wouldn't come out so I had to leave them a lot. I found it was better if two of us went, then we could talk together and he could listen without getting tired out—but this was difficult to arrange every day.'

The respondents tended to prefer free visiting hours to fixed ones,[1] but again one wonders what the people who died felt about this. They may have wanted the companionship of people near and dear to them but not necessarily to have been exposed to all the friends and relatives who chose to visit them. A few of the comments show that some respondents were aware of the possible problems created by free visiting if prospective visitors did not exercise discretion.

> 'I could have stayed the whole time if I liked but I don't think you want a crowd in a surgical ward. I felt anyway he'd just had an operation—didn't want to keep talking.'

Other comments indicate the dilemma:

> 'She had lots of friends as well as relatives. It was a case of fitting everybody in'.

Bearing the brunt

We asked the person we interviewed who they thought had borne the brunt of looking after the person who died.[2] Their replies are shown in Table 62. For 17% of the people no one was thought to have 'borne the brunt' of care. In over half of these the person had not needed any care; for some, a quarter, the care had been shared and for the remainder the care that was given at home was not felt to justify the phrase 'bearing the brunt'. 'Right up to the end he tried to do things for himself and there was very little to do for him.'

Wives and husbands generally bore the brunt of caring for the married, daughters for the widowed, sisters and other relatives for the single. People living alone were least likely to have someone taking on this role.

The people identified in this way may be compared to 'responsors'—those responding to needs and assuming responsibility—described in an American study of chronic illness.[3]

[1] The proportions who thought the arrangements were satisfactory were 82% when visiting was at set times; 93% when there was free visiting and 92% when there was some other arrangement.

[2] Question 51: 'Who would you say bore the brunt of looking after ——, you or someone else?'

[3] Golodetz, Arnold, *et al.*, 'The Care of Chronic Illness: The "Responsor" Role'.

TABLE 62 *The brunt bearers*

	Marital status of person who died			*Household composition of person who died*				*All*[b]
	Single	*Married*	*Widowed etc.*	*On own*	*With spouse only*	*With other relatives*[a]	*With unrelated people*	
	%	%	%	%	%	%	%	%
Those in same household:								
Wife	—	50	—	—	45	23	—	27
Husband	—	24	—	—	28	7	—	13
Daughter	—	3	40	—	—	33	—	16
Son	—	1	5	—	—	4	—	2
Daughter-in-law	—	—	6	—	—	4	—	2
Sister or sister-in-law	34	1	4	—	—	11	—	6
Other	27	1	4	—	—	5	66	5
Those not in same household:								
Daughter	—	2	10	23	2	2	—	5
Son	—	—	3	7	1	—	—	1
Other relative	13	1	4	16	2	1	5	3
Friend, neighbour or other person	13	—	5	17	1	1	5	3
No one	13	17	19	37	21	9	24	17
Number of deaths (=100%)	62	329	215	84	197	302	21	616

[a] With or without their spouse.
[b] Those who were in a hospital or institution for a year or more before they died and those who died unexpectedly before they were 65 have been excluded.

As in that study, the person was almost always a family member (nine-tenths), and generally a woman (three-quarters).

Of the daughters who lived in the household and had borne the brunt of care, nearly a third were unmarried. When the wives, husbands or daughters had borne the brunt of care we interviewed them personally in the majority of cases, 90%. When someone else had borne the brunt we were rather less often able to interview them—in 74% of the cases.

A third of the respondents who said they had borne the brunt were 65 or more. This proportion was 47% for both husbands and wives, 4% for sons and daughters, 54% for brothers and sisters. We asked the person we interviewed about the differences looking after the person who died had made to their lives and, if they worked, about any changes they had to make in their work. Replies are considered separately (in Table 63) for principal caregivers and for those who helped but felt that someone else had borne the main burden of care. Three-tenths of the 'brunt-bearers' we talked to had worked full-time when they started to look after the person who died.[1]

A quarter of the brunt-bearers who worked gave up working altogether in order to look after the person who died. Expressing this in terms of the number of people who gave up work per 100 people dying, the estimate is between six and nine.[2] About two-fifths of those who gave up work did so for a year or longer. The numbers whose work was affected in some way were between twenty-two and twenty-six per 100 people dying, and that does not include all the people who helped, only those we interviewed and who bore the brunt. The median length of time for which their work was affected was almost four months. Over two-fifths of those whose work had been affected said it made a lot of difference to them financially.[3]

The point most frequently made when we asked the brunt-bearers to describe any other differences looking after the dying person had made to their lives, was the effect on their social lives. Two-fifths mentioned this, and among the daughters living in the same household the proportion was three-fifths.

> One daughter who lived with her father, husband, mother-in-law and her own daughter explained: 'It's a difficult one to answer really. The whole routine changed. With a child, mother-in-law and husband you had to fit everything in. The household revolved round father. The others could at least help themselves a bit! He couldn't at all. You

[1] Question 55: 'Were you working at the time you started to look after ——?' IF YES 'Was it full or part time?'

[2] This depends on whether those who had been in hospital or institution for a year or more before they died are estimated as not having anyone who gave up work to look after them before they went into hospital or whether they are counted as being 'at risk' in the same way as others.

[3] Question 58: 'Did this [change in work] make a lot, a little or no difference to you financially?'

TABLE 63 *Effect on respondent's work*

	Respondents who bore brunt							*Other respondents*		
	Wife	*Husband*	*Daughter in same household*	*Other person in household*	*Daughter outside household*	*Other person outside household*	*All respondents who bore brunt*	*Male*	*Female*	*All respondents*
	%	%	%	%	%	%	%	%	%	%
Working:										
full-time	9	54	36	40	23	32	30	69	28	32
part-time	15	11	10	10	27	22	14	—	18	13
not at all	76	35	54	50	50	46	56	31	54	55
Number of respondents (=100%)	140	72	95	66	30	37	440	29	65	534
	%	%	%	%	% (Daughter and other person outside household combined)		%	% (Male and female combined)		%
Changes:										
To different hours	6	11	9	—	9		7	4		7
To less hours	3	19	14	13	3		11	6		10
To different work	—	4	2	9	3		4	2		3
Taking time off	29	45	42	25	43		38	34		37
Retiring early	—	2	5	—	—		2	2		2
Giving up work altogether	47	30	23	19	6		25	2		21
Other or unspecified changes	21	9	12	13	3		11	4		10
No changes	9	13	16	34	49		23	49		28
Number of respondents who were working (=100%)[a]	34	47	43	32	35		191	47		238

don't think of that at the time. You take it in your stride. You've got to.' Her father had died at home of lung cancer after being bedridden for more than three months.

Another daughter who was single and under 35 had lived just with her mother who had been ill 'ever since I was a little girl. Mind you she was always very good. She never restricted me in any way. I wasn't quite as free as a normal girl would be. I suppose it used to depress me at times. You did not consciously begrudge it. You tended to resentfulness, not consciously. I might have been going out and I'd say no, even if I was looking forward to it.'

Another single daughter who had been living just with her mother was between 55 and 65. She told us: 'I stopped working in London sixteen years ago when my father was ill, to help and to be company for my mother after he died.'

A husband who had looked after his wife during a comparatively short illness had given up his work for between one and three months. 'I only left her for about half an hour [at a time]—no longer—because when I went out I wanted to get back. If I went for a drink I didn't enjoy it.'

Another example of the effect on people's social lives came from a woman whose father-in-law had died of stomach cancer. He had come to live with her, her husband and four sons:

'It wore us out completely. We were shut in. Well it changed our whole way of living. But what is a couple of months? It made him so happy to be with us.'

A fifth of those who bore the brunt felt it had been a strain on them.

'I very rarely got a whole night's sleep. Always on the alert if he got up from a chair and stumbled. I didn't like to leave him for long in case he fell. Couldn't relax at all' (wife whose husband 'had ailed for years' but died of a cerebral thrombosis).

'It was always on your mind—you could never relax.' (A daughter-in-law who lived almost opposite her father-in-law. She had taken meals across to him for six weeks before he went into hospital where he died a fortnight later from cancer.)

'I got irritable—not very nice to live with. Last three weeks at night we were staying up—me and my daughter. Tempers were frayed with the rest of the family through no sleep. A home help would have been ideal—we would have caught up on a bit of sleep' (a daughter who lived next door to her mother).

Another daughter whose mother came to live with her, her husband and two children three years before she died described how it had affected their social lives and been a strain: 'We could never go out for very long. It got everyone in the end. We were all under such a strain. In the last few weeks we didn't have an evening to ourselves. We had no peace of mind at all. We almost lost touch with our friends as we couldn't visit them or have them here.'

Golodetz and his colleagues also described the sense of isolation in households caring for the chronically sick.[1] They also found that the health of responsers was 'surprisingly bad'. One in seven of the brunt-bearers on this study said that looking after the person who died had affected their health.

'It made me feel quite ill in myself and I don't think it was very nice for my son to have to put up with the smell and everything.' (A daughter whose father had been bedridden for over six months and doubly incontinent for over three months.)

A wife who had looked after her husband whom she described as dying 'from a diseased heart brought on by dust' said she had been 'very depressed'. He was her second husband and she had nursed her first husband for twenty-one years before he died of T.B. 'You feel some days that everything is down on you and it's not worth living. It does make you feel that way. I can't go to my children—they've enough trouble of their own.'

One in six mentioned that they had been glad to help in the way they did.

[1] Golodetz, Arnold, *et al.*, op. cit.

A woman who had helped her sister to wash and undress and lift herself up when she became bedridden and mentally confused over a month before she died described the help she gave as 'what anyone else would do. You go on, day after day.'

A friend who had known the person who died for over twenty years stayed with her for some time and helped with various personal and household things, said 'I spent a good deal of time down there and would have stayed as long as she needed me and loved to do it. We were very close. She loved me and liked to have me there.'

One in eight said it made very little difference to them.

A wife whose husband had been bedridden for less than a month before he died at home explained: 'It didn't really make much difference because he insisted on doing all he could for himself. I had to slow myself down. I'm very active and I had to slow down to his pace.'

Another wife whose husband had died of cancer said that looking after him had made no difference to her life, only 'we couldn't go out, but we've never been a gallivanting pair'.

One in seven maintained that it had not made any difference to their lives.

A wife who had helped her husband with washing, dressing, getting in and out of bed, getting to the lavatory and with other personal needs for over a year ('he'd been up and down with heart trouble for seven years') said: 'It made no difference. We were always contented together in the house whether he was well or not. Once in a blue moon when he was well we would go to the pictures but we liked it best at home.'

A woman whose cousin of 75 lived with her and her family had only helped him with one or two things in the last week of his life: 'There was no difference. He was very little trouble. We all liked him and he was very kind to us. He used to do little bits of shopping for us.'

Many of these comments reveal the sort of relationship that informants had with the person who died and give some idea of the gap that was left in their lives by their bereavement. This is discussed in more detail in Chapter 10.

Conclusions

The overwhelming impression of the data presented in this chapter is of the extent of support provided by relatives, friends and neighbours to people in the last year of their lives. A study in Glasgow reported similar findings: 'Neglect of old people by relatives played a negligible part in the demand for admission to hospital. On the contrary, the help received from relatives, who were for the most part themselves middle-aged or elderly, was vast and was given willingly and cheerfully, so long as conditions were tolerable.'[1] It is perhaps surprising that this informal network of relatives and friends seems to work in such an effective way: wives and husbands care for the married, daughters for the widowed, sisters and more distant relatives for the single. Friends and neighbours generally give less intimate types of care, but if there are no relatives to help they often step into the breach. And the more things people need help with, the more people there seem to be who rally round and help.

There are a number of problems with these types of arrangements. Earlier chapters have shown that people without close relatives to help them are more likely to be admitted to hospitals and institutions, but facilities for long-term nursing care of elderly patients are often inadequate. When places cannot be found for people who need help with self care and some nursing care over a long time an undue burden and strain is put on their relatives and friends. And some relatives and friends may lack the facilities, strength, time, patience and skills to look after people with terminal illness at home.

[1] Isaacs, Bernard, 'Geriatric patients: do their families care?'

9

AWARENESS AND INFORMATION ABOUT DEATH AND ILLNESS

Much has been written about people's awareness of dying. Their denial and acceptance, their anger, depression and hope in this circumstance have been discussed, as have the roles played by their family and by professionals in supporting them when they are faced with this realisation or in protecting them from such knowledge.[1]

Studies of dying patients and their awareness of death have inevitably been confined to special groups suffering from recognised terminal illness.[2] Our study, covering a sample of all deaths, depends on the reports and perceptions of relatives. We do not know with any certainty whether the person who died realised he was dying; relatives told us whether they thought the person knew this.[3] Our information relates to relatives' awareness and views about the knowledge both they and the person who died had at the time. We also asked the general practitioners, district nurses and health visitors in our study for their views about handling questions from dying patients about their prognosis.

The extent of awareness

Table 64 shows how far the respondents thought they themselves and the people who died were aware of what was wrong

[1] See Brauer, P. H., 'Should the patient be told the truth?'; Glaser, Barney G. and Strauss, Anselm L., *Awareness of Dying*; Hinton, John, *Dying*; Kubler-Ross, Elisabeth, *On Death and Dying*; Pearson, Leonard (ed.), *Death and Dying*.

[2] Exton-Smith, A. N., 'Terminal illness in the aged'; Wilkes, E., 'Terminal cancer at home'.

[3] In this chapter those under 65 who died unexpectedly with no previous restriction have been excluded. We have also excluded respondents who were not relatives or close friends of the person who died. This has reduced the sample first from 785 to 727 and then to 686.

(the condition) and what was likely to happen (the outcome). It also shows their sources of information about this. According to the respondents, almost half of the people who died knew what was wrong with them,[1] a third did not know, and for the remaining 17% the respondents were uncertain.

TABLE 64 *Knowledge of dying person's condition and outcome and source of information*

	Dying person's knowledge of		*Respondent's knowledge of*	
	Condition	*Outcome*	*Condition*	*Outcome*
	%	%	%	%
Knew	49	37	83	73
Did not know	34	43	10	18
Half knew/Uncertain	17	20	7	9
Knew—told by	%[a]	%[a]	%[a]	%[a]
No one	11	31	6	9
General practitioner	28	3	47	36
Hospital doctor	10	2	23	22
Hospital sister/nurse	—	—	5	7
Dying person[b]	—	—	3	—
Other	3	1	6	5
Number of deaths (=100%)	682	691	667	649

[a] Percentages may add to more than the total who knew since it was possible for information to come from more than one source.
[b] This answer was recorded only for the source of the respondent's information on the dying person's condition.

Fewer were thought to have known that they were unlikely to recover.[2] Thirty-seven per cent were thought to have known either probably or certainly; 43% probably or definitely did not know, and for 20% the respondents were unable to say whether the dying person knew or not. We cannot tell how often the person who died knew what was wrong or that he was dying but did not reveal this to the respondent. If we

[1] Question 65: 'Did —— know what was wrong with him?'
[2] Question 66: 'Did —— know he was not likely to recover?' or 'Did —— know this was likely to happen?'

exclude the uncertain answers we find that, according to our respondents, 47% of our subjects probably or definitely knew. This finding is similar to Hinton's[1] estimate of the extent to which dying patients in a general hospital knew they were dying. He found that 18% spoke of death as a possibility, 26% were more sure of death and 6% were unhesitating about it; that is half of them might have known to some degree.

A higher proportion of the respondents said they themselves knew both about the condition and the probable outcome.[2] Eighty-three per cent said they knew what was wrong and 73% said they knew what the outcome would be. But even though three-quarters of the respondents said they knew that the person was going to die, only a fifth expected him to die at the time when he did.[3] Fourteen per cent expected the person to die earlier, 15% were uncertain and 24% expected him to die later. For example, this man knew his wife was going to die but expected her to die later:

> 'I knew from the onset, the first attack, that one day one would finish her. I didn't have to ask the doctor. It is preferable to face up to reality. I certainly wasn't expecting it at that time as she had been fit over Christmas.'

The length of time for which the outcome was known is shown in Table 65. Rather less than half of the people who died and half of the respondents who knew had known for three months or more.

General practitioners were the main source of information about the condition for both the respondents and the people who died and about the outcome for the respondents. But the respondents thought that most of the people who knew they were dying had not been told by anyone.

> 'He was that sort of man—he liked to know. In the last few weeks he said, "Something's happening to my body that's strange", so he must have felt bad then. A week

[1] Hinton, op. cit., pp. 95–6.

[2] Question 67: 'What about from your point of view. Did you know what was wrong with ——?' Question 68: 'I think you said you: knew/didn't know/half knew that —— was unlikely to recover?'

[3] Question 68(d): 'Did you expect —— to die earlier, later or when he did?'

TABLE 65 *Length of time the person who died and respondent knew outcome*

	How long person who died knew outcome[a]	*How long respondent knew outcome*[b]
	%	%
Less than a week	18	17
A week or more but less than 3 months	38	34
3 months or more	44	49
Numbers of dying people or respondents who knew (=100%)	204	446

[a] Question 66(c): 'How long before he died had he (or might he have) known?'
[b] Question 68(b): 'How long had you known before he died?'

before [he died] he said "I think I'm finished now".' (This man's wife said he knew certainly he was dying, but no one had told him.)

'I think inwardly she knew that the end was coming.' (This woman 'probably' knew, but no one had told her.)

The respondents were more likely to have received information from all sources than the people who died. Three per cent of the respondents reported that they found out what was wrong from the dying person himself. There did not seem to be any such information passing from the respondent to the person who died.

'She told me she would die suddenly. I hoped she would recover. Didn't know she was going to [die].'

'She often said she wouldn't live long and I didn't take her seriously until she began to deteriorate.'

There were also some respondents who thought that people did not know they were dying although they knew what was wrong with them.

'She knew she had a stroke but she didn't know she was not likely to recover.'

Other people probably knew they were dying but had not been told what was wrong with them, as the following report from a woman whose husband died in hospital of cancer shows.

'I think in the end he did know, the way he kept looking at me. He said to me "I've gone thinner since I came in". And I said, "It's imagination", but he said, "No". '

Relatives' views[1]

Relatives' views on whether it was better for themselves and the people who died to know the outcome are shown in Table 66.[2]

As might be expected, most of the relatives thought it was 'best as it was' except when they themselves did not know what was likely to happen.

Relatives' views about the dying person's knowledge were the reverse of those about their own knowledge. They tended to believe it was better if the dying person did not know, but better for themselves to know. In 82% of the instances where the people who died did not know the probable outcome, the relatives thought this was best. A similar proportion of the relatives, 86%, thought it best as it was when they themselves knew the prognosis. Only 2% of those who said the dying person did not know thought it would have been better if he had done so. Table 67 summarises their views on this.

Many of the relatives had strong feelings on these points. Some thought that if the person had known about his impending death this might have hastened it.

'If he had known he would have gone sooner. He was fighting all the time.' (This man died of cancer.)

[1] In fact the views are those of our respondents—excluding unrelated people who were not close friends of the person who died. Ninety-five per cent were relatives.

[2] For example, Question 66(b): 'Do you think that was best or do you think it would have been better if he had not known (or had known definitely)?', and Question 68(c): 'Would you have preferred not to know or do you think it was better that you did?'

TABLE 66 *Respondents' views of their and dead person's knowledge of outcome*

	Knowledge of outcome				
	Person who died definitely or probably did not know	*Person who died certainly or probably knew*	*Respondent did not know*	*Respondent half knew*	*Respondent knew*
Respondents' assessment of what was best:	%	%	%	%	%
Better to have known (definitely)	2	8	43	22	—
Better not to have known (definitely)	9	17	—	7	4
Best as it was	82	55	48	62	86
Uncertain	7	20	9	9	10
Number of people who died or respondents (=100%)	287	247	111	55	456

TABLE 67 *Respondents' assessment of best state of awareness*

	Best for person who died	*Best for respondent*
	%	%
Best/better to have known (definitely)	24	73
Best/better not to have known	45	12
Half knew—that was best	—	5
Qualified, uncertain[a]	31	10
Number of respondents (=100%)	669	621

[a] This figure includes the 20% of whom the respondents were unsure whether or not they knew the outcome.

> 'I pretended it was ulcers and I got the hospital doctor to say the same. I didn't want her to know. If she'd known, she'd have gone straight through the door and finished it. She was like that.' (This man's wife also died of cancer.)

It seemed that a number of the relatives, like this man, were prepared to assume responsibility for the dying person, and withhold the truth from them. Another study found similar collusion between the relatives and doctors of dying patients.

> 'In 73% of the 37 expected deaths, a mutual decision was made by the physician and the family to avoid letting the sick person know the truth about his condition and its expected outcome.'[1]

It is not possible to estimate the proportion of people in our study whose relatives and doctors came to a mutual decision not to tell. But from comments such as these from relatives, and the responses of doctors, which we examine later, it is clear that this sort of practice was quite common.

Apart from a fear of the patient committing suicide, other relatives indicated that if the dying person had known about the outcome he would have been more worried or depressed.

> 'She did get very upset about things and she'd have got more depressed if she had known.' (This woman died of congestive heart failure after being an invalid for over eight months.)

> 'He would have worried that much over my mother, it would have been too much of a strain. It was bad enough my mother having to put on an act.' (This man's father died of cancer, deteriorating rapidly in the last two weeks. He lived with his wife only.)

It is likely that some strain was put on the relationships between the people who died and their relatives as a result of the pretence the relatives felt they had to maintain. One man told us of the dilemma he found himself in when he was told his wife had cancer, but did not let her know.

[1] Duff, Raymond S. and Hollingshead, August B., *Sickness and Society*, p. 310.

'The nurse came along as I was sitting at my wife's bedside and told me Mr P. wanted to speak to me. My wife immediately asked "Why?" I said to my wife, "I don't know what he wants." I went out and saw Mr P. and he broke the news that my wife had cancer. My wife had asked me to go back and tell what he'd said. So I said to Mr P., "What am I to tell my wife?" He was very off hand about the whole thing. He couldn't have cared less what I should say. I then spoke to the nurse and asked her. She suggested I should say they wanted to know whether there was a 'phone at home. Finally I decided to tell her that they'd enquired about facilities at home and that's how I got out of it. I do think the nurse could have been more tactful.'

This is an example of what Glaser and Strauss have called 'closed awareness';[1] the management by relatives and professionals of the information given to the patient in order to prevent him from becoming aware.

Hinton found that 'only a minority of marital partners had spoken to each other explicitly in a way that indicated they both acknowledged that one of them might shortly die.'[2] And Abrams thinks most terminal cancer patients opt for denial of dying as a response to their worsening condition.[3] In her view the non-communication is a source of strain on the relationships between the dying person and his caregivers. She holds the view that 'the latter should not fight these defences', but should adapt to them for the patient's sake, and maintain a mutual pretence. Saunders, on the other hand, has described the help and support given at one hospital to both patients and families so that there can often be a sharing of awareness and a consequent relaxation of tension.[4] Our findings suggest that many people who are dying are not told that this is happening. They are not given the opportunity to accept it or deny it. Most of those who were thought to be aware of it had apparently reached this conclusion on their own.

[1] Glaser and Strauss, *Awareness of Dying,* pp. 29–46.

[2] Hinton, John, 'Communication between husband and wife in terminal cancer'.

[3] Abrams, R. D., 'The defences of the terminal cancer patient'.

[4] Saunders, Cicely M. S., 'The moment of truth: care of the dying person'.

Sometimes relatives felt that when the person realised he was dying he had gone downhill as a result. For example, a woman told of her husband who probably knew he was dying:

> 'I think towards the very end, he knew. I could tell he was giving way. If he'd known a year ago, he wouldn't have lived, especially if he'd known he had cancer. He had a horror of that.'

In some cases where the person knew, it was taken quite calmly, as by the woman whose husband felt it was best that she knew that she had heart trouble and would probably die.

> 'Well aware and accepted it. She was a brave woman willing to face up to facts. Travelled the world with me, was used to accepting things as she found them.'

Most of the relatives who knew what was going to happen expressed the opinion that it was best that they knew because they were able to prepare themselves.

> 'I think it's best—why build up hope? It's more of a shock then.'

> 'You know how to act when you actually get in the hospital. You could cheer him up, but seeing him get lower and lower you might have said something to worry him if you did not already know.'

Some respondents who did not know thought it would have been better if they had known, for similar reasons. One woman whose mother died of heart failure would have liked to have known because 'I could have stopped work to have had more time with her'.

And a man whose wife died in hospital said:

> 'I would have stayed up near the hospital and spent more time with her.'

These relatives were of course giving us their views about what happened in this particular experience of theirs. Their feelings about whether it was better for either themselves or the person who was dying to have known what was happening will have been affected not only by that experience but also by their previous expectations of what is appropriate in such situations and they will also be influenced by the ethos of doctors and other professionals they came into contact with at that time. In addition they live in a society which tends to regard death as a taboo subject.[1]

Information about the illness

Relatives were also asked if they were able to find out all they wanted to know about the illness or incapacity of the person who died and how it was likely to affect him.[2] Twenty-four per cent said they were not. A further 5% would have liked something explained in more detail, and 4% were not able to find out about things as soon as they wanted to. The remaining 67% were able to find out all they wanted to, in as much detail, and as soon as they wanted.

In some cases the respondents knew all they wanted to because they had been given the information.

> 'They told me directly as soon as she was taken in.' (This man's wife was taken into hospital and he was told right away that she had cancer.)

For some little or no information was needed.

> 'I knew when they took her that she would not come back. There wasn't anything to find out, she was unconscious.' (This woman's mother had a stroke and was taken to hospital where she died soon after.)

Other respondents knew all that they wanted to, although they clearly did not know all there was to know and admitted this.

> 'The sister in hospital asked me if I knew what was wrong. She said it had turned to cancer. They didn't give me much information. They just drifted on. But I didn't want to know more.'

What about that third of the respondents who were not fully

[1] See Gorer, Geoffrey, *Death, Grief and Mourning in Contemporary Britain*, p. 172.

[2] Question 60: 'During ——'s illness or incapacity were you able to find out all you wanted to know about his illness and how it was likely to affect him?' *If Yes*: 'Was there anything else you would have liked to have explained to you in more detail?' *If No*: 'Were you able to find out about things as soon as you wanted to?'

informed? Altogether 13% of the respondents did not ask anyone for more or earlier information, as in the case of this respondent.[1]

> 'The doctor used to tell my sister [person who died] about her illness. I just used to wonder why these strokes attacked her but I didn't ask anybody.'

Although the remaining 20% asked someone about what they wanted to know, only 7% reported that they were given additional information on asking.

> 'Really I knew nothing until the doctor at the hospital told me. Eventually it was all explained and I realised nothing on earth could help him. If we'd really known what was wrong—if I'd had an inkling—they gave me nothing. I asked my own doctor and he could only say what they'd told him at the hospital, when he started going to out-patients' (her husband died of cancer).

Half of those who asked for more information consulted a general practitioner, a quarter asked a hospital doctor, and a quarter asked a hospital sister or nurse; one in eight asked someone else. Even when the person had died in a hospital or institution the general practitioner was still the person from whom relatives most often sought information: just over two-fifths had asked him while about a third had talked to a hospital sister or nurse and slightly fewer to a doctor at the hospital. A third of those who asked said they were given more information.

Whether or not relatives had all the information they wanted was closely related to their knowledge of what was wrong with the person who died and what was likely to happen. This is shown in Table 68. The association is more marked with the respondent's knowledge of the condition than with knowledge of the outcome.

Sources of information

Table 69 shows the professionals to whom relatives had talked

[1] Question 62: 'Did you ask anyone about this?' *If Yes*: (a) 'Whom did you ask?' (b) 'What happened?'

TABLE 68 *Adequacy of information and knowledge of condition and outcome*

	Respondent's knowledge of condition			*Respondent's knowledge of outcome*		
	Knew	*Half knew*	*Did not know*	*Knew*	*Half knew*	*Did not know*
	%	%	%	%	%	%
Respondent found out all wanted to, in as much detail and as soon as wanted	74	33	27	75	56	41
Respondent would have liked more/more detailed/earlier information	26	67	73	25	44	59
Number of respondents (=100%)	511	39	51	451	54	103

about the dead person's illness and about what was likely to happen.[1]

General practitioners were again the main source of information except when the person who died had been in hospital for a year or more, when it was a hospital sister or nurse.[2] Five per cent of those said to have given most information were not professional people but other relatives.

Some relatives had found it difficult to get information from the hospital. They did not know who to approach and those they talked to were evasive.

> 'I found the hospital very unapproachable, our own doctor was much better.'

> 'He [general practitioner] can't tell you till he gets reports from hospital. Hospitals don't give you straight answers. They beat about the bush.'

> 'G.P. gave some information but not enough. Hospital was

[1] Question 63: 'Who did you talk to about ——'s illness and what was likely to happen?'

[2] Question 64(a): 'Who gave you most information?'

TABLE 69 *Discussion about illness and outcome with professionals by how long person who died was in hospital in last year of life*

	Length of time person who died was in hospital during the last year of life				
	Not at all	*Less than a month*	*A month but less than a year*	*A year or more*	*All*
	%	%	%	%	%
Dead person's general practitioner	76	69	63	48	67
Other general practitioner	14	11	9	11	11
Hospital doctor	15	45	52	41	39
Hospital sister or nurse	3	36	49	65	33
District nurse	18	8	13	4	12
Clergyman	11	8	11	9	10
Other professional	7	7	11	37	10
No professional	13	10	5	2	9
Number of respondents (=100%)	169	213	195	46	635

worse. No information whatever from hospital, not very enlightening—couldn't contact people to find things out.'

All of these respondents said that they had been given most information by a general practitioner.

Hospital sisters and nurses were quite a frequent source of information, as in this case:

'I didn't know what was wrong until they took an X-ray. The sister said, "How much do you know?" I said, "I'm not sure. The male nurse said it might be cancer." She said, "It is cancer. He can't last much longer." '

Although a third of the people who died had been visited at home by district nurses during their last year and one in eight of the relatives had discussed the illness with them, only 3% of the respondents said the district nurse gave them most information.

Factors related to levels of information

People dying from cancer were less likely to have known what was wrong with them than those dying from other diseases. At least, that was the view of their relatives who reckoned that 29% of those who died from cancer knew what was wrong compared with 57% of those dying from other diseases. The dead person's general practitioner was the most frequent source of this information in all but the cancer deaths: 34% of the people who died from other causes were said to have been told what was wrong by their doctor; this was only 7% for those with cancer. Hospital doctors did not make up for this deficit, although those dying of cancer were more likely to have been in hospital. Twelve per cent of those dying from cancer were said to have known what was wrong although no one had told them explicitly.

The information about what was wrong was thought to have been withheld effectively from half the patients who died from cancer. It was not withheld from most of the relatives we interviewed, as can be seen from the second part of Table 70. For them a hospital doctor was a relatively frequent source of information when the person died of cancer.

It appears from these results that doctors treat the information that a patient has cancer in much the same way as they treat information about his impending death: they conceal it from him but tell his relatives.

The longer a person had been ill and the more severely restricted he was, the more likely both he and his relatives were to realise that he was dying. This is shown in Table 71. Physical clues are obviously important in determining awareness. For example 79% of those persons who were said to have known they were going to die suffered from pain compared with 70% of those said not to know.

Older people were no more likely than younger ones to know that they might die, according to their relatives. But our respondents themselves were less likely to have known that the person was going to die if he was 65 or more years old than if he was younger: 70% compared with 81%.

It might be expected that the closer a relative was to a person the more likely he would be to know that the person

TABLE 70 *Knowledge of what was wrong and source of this information for those dying of cancer and other diseases*

	Cause of death	
a) *Dead person's knowledge of his condition*	*Neoplasms*	*Other*
	%	%
Dead person did not know what was wrong	49	27
Uncertain	22	16
Dead person knew what was wrong	29	57
Told by:[a]	%	%
General practitioner	7	34
Hospital doctor	8	10
Other person	3	3
No one	12	10
Number of deaths (=100%)[b]	204	478
b) *Respondent's knowledge of dead person's condition*	*Neoplasms*	*Other*
	%	%
Respondent did not know	8	10
Respondent half knew	4	8
Respondent knew	88	82
Told by:[a]	%	%
General practitioner	43	48
Hospital doctor	41	15
Hospital sister/nurse	4	6
Dead person	2	3
Other	6	7
No one	3	7
Number of deaths (=100%)[b]	202	465

[a] Percentages may add to more than the total who were told because more than one person may have given them this information.

[b] Small numbers for whom inadequate information was obtained have been omitted when calculating percentages.

TABLE 71 *Respondent's and dead person's knowledge of outcome and dead person's restrictions*

Summary of restrictions	*Proportion of people who died who probably or certainly knew*		*Proportion of respondents who knew the outcome*	
Bedridden for more than 3 months	49%	(78)	89%	(75)
Confined to bed or severely restricted for more than 3 months	43%	(204)	80%	(189)
Other restrictions for more than 3 months	37%	(215)	68%	(210)
All restrictions for less than 3 months	28%	(120)	70%	(108)
No restrictions	21%	(58)	50%	(52)
All deaths	37%	(675)	73%	(634)

The figures in brackets are the numbers on which the percentages are based (=100%).

was dying. In fact Table 72 shows that husbands and wives were less likely than other relatives to say they knew that the deceased was going to die, while sons or daughters were the most likely to know.[1] A patient's husband or wife may be the last person to 'give up hope'. In the same way that they deny the existence of certain unpleasant symptoms,[2] they may reject the idea that death is imminent or inevitable. Sons and daughters of the person who died were also more likely to find out all they wanted to know than other respondents, 74% compared with 64%.

When the person died in a hospital or other institution rather than in his own or someone else's home there was no difference in the extent of his or the respondent's knowledge of the condition or outcome. However, when people died in hospital respondents were less likely to have all the information they would have liked, 63% compared with 72%.

[1] See also Appendix V: 'Data from different types of respondents'.
[2] See Appendix V.

TABLE 72 *Respondent's awareness of outcome by relationship to person who died*

Respondent's knowledge of the outcome:	*Respondent's relationship to person who died*			
	Husband or wife	*Son or daughter*	*Other relative*	*Unrelated person*
	%	%	%	%
Knew the person was unlikely to recover	68	78	75	70
Half knew the person was unlikely to recover	10	8	8	7
Did not know the person was unlikely to recover	22	14	17	23
Number of respondents (=100%)	252	225	142	30

Professionals' views

Saunders had argued that in caring for the dying 'the real question is not, "What do you tell your patients?", but rather, "What do you let your patients tell you?" '[1] Our question to general practitioners was less subtle. We asked what they would do when confronted with cancer patients who would almost certainly die within six weeks but whose circumstances and response to the situation varied in different ways.[2] Their replies are shown in Table 73.

Doctors were most likely to say they would tell the truth to the businessman of 55 who asks directly. Two-thirds felt they would do so in this situation but one in four would either deny that a person was dying or evade the question. Nine per cent gave qualified answers which were sometimes related to the extent of the man's responsibilities.

'I've never had to do it. If the man has just a small business,

[1] Saunders, Cicely, 'The moment of truth: care of the dying person', p. 59.

[2] They were asked specifically about cancer patients because it was thought that this was a disease for which it was sometimes realistic for doctors to say people 'will almost certainly die within six weeks'.

TABLE 73 *What the doctor would do in different situations*

What the doctor would probably do in these situations[a]	*People with cancer who will almost certainly die within six weeks*		
	Businessman of 55 who asks 'Is this going to kill me, doctor?'	*Young mother of 35 with young children who does not raise subject and seems unaware*	*Elderly widower who asks 'This won't kill me doctor, will it?'*
	%	%	%
Tell person the truth	65	2	13
Tell their spouse the truth	—	97	—
Say he does not know	10	—	—
Deny that they will die	12	—	39
Pass it off as a joke, change subject	4	—	34
Qualified answer	9	1	14
Number of doctors (=100%)		323[b]	

[a] Question 25: 'Whether a person should be told that they are dying probably depends on a number of different things. But could you say what you would probably do in these situations—all related to people with cancer who will almost certainly die within six weeks?'

[b] Small numbers for whom inadequate answers were obtained have been omitted in calculating percentages.

not much responsibility, I would tell him a lie, but if the man had a great many responsibilities, I would probably tell him.'

The reason most frequently given for telling the businessman who asked directly was so that he could put his affairs in order.

'I believe it to be utterly wrong, even impertinent to deny a responsible man the right to "put his house in order".'

Few seemed to feel that if people ask they have a right to be told the truth whatever their situation. But a number said they had never been asked.

'I've never told a patient yet that they're going to die, and I've never been asked. If I was asked by a businessman with commitments I would tell him.'

Only 2% said they would tell a young mother with young children who seemed unaware, but most, 98%, said they would tell her husband. Rather more, 13%, would tell the elderly widower the truth when he asked the loaded question. But the majority would not and some were emphatic about this.

'I wouldn't tell him. I told two of mine and they committed suicide by putting their heads in the gas oven.'

'It would be quite impossible to tell any patient personally—I would *never* tell *any* patient in *any* circumstances that they were dying of cancer. I should lie like a trooper to the last minute.'

It seemed in general that most doctors felt they would protect their patients' interests by telling those with financial or business responsibilities who asked directly that they would die. When people had family responsibilities and did not ask they would not tell them but would tell some other responsible person.

These findings and the relatives' estimates of whether people knew they were dying are rather similar to results from American studies which showed that 'sixty to ninety per cent of doctors (depending on the study) favour not telling their patients about terminal illness'.[1] Glaser and Strauss compare this with 'the ideal rule offered by doctors that in each individual case they should decide whether the patient really wants to know and can "take it"'. They conclude:

'It appears that most doctors have a general standard from which the same decision flows for most patients—that they should not be told. This finding also indicates that the standard of "do not tell" receives very strong support from colleagues.'

We asked the district nurses and health visitors what they would do if a dying patient asked them about his prognosis. Their replies are shown in Table 74 alongside the views of general

[1] Glaser and Strauss, *Awareness of Dying*, p. 119.

practitioners on what they would like district nurses to do in such a situation.

Over half the nurses and the doctors opted for giving hope. One nurse in seventeen felt it was appropriate for them to tell the patient the truth; rather more would evade the question by

TABLE 74 *What district nurses and health visitors would do and what general practitioners would like them to do if a dying patient asked about his prognosis*

	What district nurses and health visitors said they would do[a]	*What general practitioners would like district nurses to do*[b]
	%	%
Change subject	9	4
Tell him to ask the doctor	31	49
Tell him the truth gently	6	9
Give him hope	56	58
Qualified answer	12	22
Number of professionals (=100%)[c]	581	317

[a] Question 16: 'As a general rule, if a dying patient asked you about his prognosis which of the following would you do?'

[b] Question 26: 'As a general rule, if a dying patient asked his district nurse about his prognosis which of the following would you like her to do?'

[c] Percentages add to more than 100 as a number gave more than one answer, usually telling the person to ask their doctor as well as doing something else.

changing the subject. A greater proportion of doctors than of nurses were in favour of the nurse telling the patient to ask the doctor. It would seem that most of the nurses did 'give him hope' or referred him to his doctor, if they were ever asked by the patients in our study.

> (Give him hope) 'I want somebody to do that for me. I wouldn't want anyone to tell me I was dying so I won't do that for anyone else' (district nurse).

'I'm a bit of a coward. Who am I to take all hope away from them?' (district nurse).

'Depends on person really. Usually advise doctor. It is not our place to tell them, we've had this drilled into us. But I feel that if a person asks me outright they should be told they're dying. They should be given time to put things in order' (qualified answer by district nurse).

Both the general practitioners and the nurses were asked who they thought was usually the best person to tell a patient he was unlikely to recover. Table 75 shows that the majority of both groups thought it should be his own doctor but rather more of the doctors than the nurses thought this.

District nurses and health visitors who were attached to a general medical practice were more likely than those who were not attached to say that the doctor was the best person to tell a dying patient, 82% compared with 75%. Unattached nurses and health visitors were more likely to name other people such

TABLE 75 *General practitioners' and district nurses' views on the best person to tell a dying patient his prognosis*[a]

	District nurses and health visitors	*General practi-tioners*
	%	%
His own doctor	79	89
Another doctor	2	5
Vicar, priest or minister	15	11
Spouse	12	7
Other close relative	4	3
Nurse	2	—
Other	1	—
No one	—	1
Qualified answer	17	4
Number of professionals (=100%)[b]	577	316

[a] Question 17/27: 'If a patient is to be told that he is unlikely to recover who do you think is usually the best person to tell him?'

[b] Percentages may add to more than 100% as it was possible for more than one person to be recorded as the best person to tell.

as a vicar or priest. Fifteen per cent of the district nurses and health visitors and 11% of the doctors said that a member of the clergy was an appropriate person for this task.

> 'If he is a religious man the vicar. It wouldn't be so bad; he would find certain words to put it in a kinder way' (unattached district nurse).

> 'This depends on the person but I should say vicar or priest could offer most help' (unattached health visitor).

Only one of the subjects had been told of his impending death by a clergyman although a third of the people who died had been visited at home by a vicar, priest or minister. It would seem that this is a role which some other professional people expect the clergy to adopt, but one which they do not accept or are not given the opportunity to carry out in practice. Similarly, although 12% of nurses and health visitors and 7% of doctors thought that it may be appropriate for a spouse to tell a patient he is dying, according to our respondents less than 1% of the dying had been told this by their husband or wife.

Summary and conclusions

The major drawback in our data for this chapter is that we do not know how much the people who died knew but did not communicate to their relatives. Other studies have rather similar drawbacks. Even those based on interviews with dying patients cannot appropriately or usefully ask, 'Do you know you are dying?' So although our findings seem reasonably comparable with theirs we still do not know how far any of the studies give a true account of the dying person's awareness.

Half the relatives we interviewed said the dying person knew what was wrong and 37% that he knew that he was dying, while 83% of the relatives said they themselves knew what was wrong and 73% that he was likely to die. The relatives received more information from all sources than did the people who died. They tended to believe that it was better for the person not to know he was dying but better that they themselves should know. But 24% of the relatives said they were not able to find out all they wanted to know about the patient's illness or incapacity and how it was likely to affect him. They were less likely to have had all the information they wanted when the patient died in hospital than when he died at home and in both circumstances their main sources of information were general practitioners.

General practitioners and nurses involved in the care of terminally ill patients mostly agreed with the relatives that it was better for the dying person not to know. Some studies have suggested that the knowledge of his illness or prognosis may be likely to make a patient take action to end his life sooner.[1] However, Hinton reported that in his experience most people have reacted calmly to the knowledge of their death and some have felt better for it.[2] One study revealed that about four-fifths of patients would like to be told that they have a fatal illness.[3]

Others tend to reinforce this belief.[4] It may be that people involved in care feel it would be less distressing both for themselves and the patient if he does not know he is dying. But they may feel this only because they do not know how to cope with the idea of death. This may apply as much to doctors and nurses as relatives. It seems there is a conspiracy of silence about death, not only among professionals.

[1] Jones, K., 'Suicide and the hospital service'; Sainsbury, Peter, *Suicide in London*; Seager, C. P. and Flood, R. A., 'Suicide in Bristol'.

[2] Hinton, J., *Dying*, p. 137.

[3] Gilbertsen, V. A. and Wangensteen, O. H., 'Should the doctor tell the patient that the disease is cancer?'

[4] Kelly, W. D. and Freissen, S. R., 'Do cancer patients want to be told?'

10

DEATH AND BEREAVEMENT

This chapter focuses on events around the time of death. It is concerned with the actual circumstances of death and what had to be done after the death. It looks at the support the surviving relatives and friends received and what support professionals felt should be given, and then considers the extent to which the bereaved had adjusted to their new state and come to terms with their loss.

Care at the time of death

Just over half (53%) of the people who died in their own or other people's homes had been seen by a general practitioner in the twenty-four hours before their death. A further quarter (26%) had been seen within the last week, 10% in the last month and 5% within the last three months. Two per cent had seen a general practitioner in the last year but not in the last three months, and 4% had not seen one for more than a year.

When the death was expected the great majority, 92%, of those dying at home had been seen by a general practitioner within the last week. The proportion was 39% for those whose death was unexpected and 70% for the intermediate group. In general, the more likely the patient was to die, in terms of age, condition and so on, the more recently he had been seen by a general practitioner. Seventy-two per cent of those dying at home of cancer had seen a general practitioner the day before they died compared with 58% of those dying at home from respiratory conditions and 41% from circulatory diseases. Eighty-four per cent of the people who died at home after having been in hospital had seen their doctor in the week before they died.

District nurses and health visitors who were giving care to people in the study were asked about the number of times they had visited the patient in the week before death.[1] Only 7% had not visited at all; 64% had been seven or more times.

Rather more of those who died in a hospital or institution than of those who died at home were said to have been unconscious when they died: two-thirds compared with just over half. This may reflect the extent to which people in hospital were under sedation or had their pain controlled. But among those who died of cancer, the cause of death most frequently associated with pain, similar proportions of those dying at home and in hospital had been unconscious.

The proportion who could always recognise relatives until they died or became unconscious was 87% of those dying at home, 75% of those dying in hospital and 64% of those dying in other institutions.[2] Those who were mentally confused were less likely to be able to recognise relatives than others, 66% compared with 89%.

Saunders has described the importance of people who are dying not feeling alone at the time of death and of 'good-byes' from the point of view of both patients and their families.[3] Eighty-seven per cent of those who died at home had relatives or friends with them at the time, and for those in hospital or institution the proportion was 24%. The overall proportion was 53%.[4] A number of our respondents described the circumstances which led to their absence at that time:

> A woman whose husband was admitted to hospital two days before he died had stayed the night at the hospital. 'At three o'clock in the morning matron said "You must come away and sleep". I didn't want to. He knew me. I said "He'll know I've gone". She insisted. She made me rest—said "You've got all day tomorrow. You mustn't loose your stamina. They'll let you know if you're

[1] Question 9(e): 'What about the last week—how many visits did he have then?' As we showed in Chapter 6, the care which these district nurses and health visitors are describing is somewhat biased in that they probably had better recall for those patients who received most care.

[2] Question 70: 'Could he recognise his relatives up until the time he died—when he was conscious?'

[3] Saunders, Cicely M. S., 'The moment of truth: care of the dying person'.

[4] This is different from the finding reported by Gorer: 'Most people, it would seem, now die alone, except for medical attendants.' See Gorer, Geoffrey, *Death, Grief and Mourning in Contemporary Britain*, p. 19.

> wanted." She made me go to bed in a women's ward. They told me at 6.15 he'd gone.'
>
> And a man whose wife died three days after she was admitted to hospital said: 'We went out for a bit of dinner and while we were gone she died.'

People who lived alone were far more likely to die alone than other people who died at home, 53% compared with 9%. Looking at it from the viewpoint of the people we interviewed, husbands and wives were with their spouse at the time of death in 94% of the cases when the person died at home, 25% when they died in hospital.[1] Comparable proportions for the sons and daughters we talked to were 82% and 22%. There were no class differences such as those found by Gorer.[2]

A death in the home

What do relatives and friends do when someone dies at home? The patient's problems end with his death, but then a new set of problems faces his survivors. The relatives must dispose of the body and see to all the formalities and rites that a death involves. There are certain legal requirements to be met before the body can be disposed of. The doctor who was looking after the person during his final illness, or the coroner, has to issue a medical certificate of the cause of death. The death must then be registered in the district where the death occurred and the registrar must issue a death certificate and disposal certificate. Once this has been done the body can be buried or cremated, and more forms have to be filled in and exchanged. Then there are further formalities to be seen to.[3] All this may have to be done by close relatives who are emotionally involved and may not be familiar with what they should do when someone dies.

When the person had died at home we asked the relatives and close friends we interviewed if they felt they knew enough

[1] Question 71: 'Were you with —— when he died?'

[2] Gorer, op. cit., p. 19.

[3] For example, the dead person's medical care, pension books, etc., must be returned to the relevant authorities, not to mention any further legal complications of insurances, wills and the like. See the Consumers' Association pamphlet, *What to do when someone dies.*

at the time about what to do when someone died at home.[1] Seventeen per cent said they would have liked to have known more. Just over half, 54%, said that they knew from experience what to do. Women over 65 seemed more likely than others to have known from experience and fewer of them would have liked to know more. Fourteen per cent of the respondents said they knew all they wanted to because they were not really involved or did not have to do anything. The other 15% had been given advice about what to do by relatives and friends, the doctor, or someone else.

For the relative of a dying person the obvious thing to do, when some crisis develops or they think the person is dying or has just died, is to call the doctor. Although the doctor may be familiar with the pattern of events leading up to death, relatives may not be, or may be alarmed and call for medical help. Some respondents found that the doctors did not like being called out in the middle of the night to attend to patients whom they knew were dying or believed to be already dead.

> 'I called the doctor after a bad night. I thought he was dying. Doctor finally came at 8.30 a.m. and was annoyed—said he *was* dying and next time to call undertaker not him.' (This woman's husband died of stomach cancer after being ill for over a year. The incident above was the last time the doctor called; he did not visit after the death at all.)

> 'She fell down the stairs but I didn't hear her. The blood was all over the place. When I found out she was out of bed I went down. The place was plastered with blood. I called the doctor but he wouldn't come. My neighbour got the police and an ambulance. We waited from 3 a.m. to 5 a.m. for the ambulance. The hospital played merry hell with me for not getting her there sooner because she was bleeding all the time.'

The medical certificate of the cause of death must be signed by the dead person's general practitioner or some other doctor attending him, unless the death is notified to the coroner in

[1] Question 77: 'Looking back on it do you think it would have been helpful if you had known more about what to do when someone died or do you feel you knew enough?' (If knew enough): 'Had someone told you about it—or did you know from previous experience?'

which case an inquiry and possibly a post-mortem may be held. Unless the relatives are uncertain whether the patient is dead there may be no need for the doctor to come to see the body if the death is expected. If the doctor has not seen the deceased person within the two weeks previous to his death he has to see the body or notify the death to the coroner.

In some cases the doctor came soon after being called when the patient gave some signs that he might be dying or that a particular crisis was developing.

> 'His wife heard a gurgling noise and went into the bedroom and thought he was dead. She rushed out to the telephone across the road to phone the doctor. When the emergency doctor came he was already dead.'

A general practitioner had come to see the person after he died in all but 8% of the home deaths. For two-thirds it was the person's own doctor, for a fifth another doctor who had seen him before, and for the remainder another doctor altogether. In 84% of cases the doctor who visited after death signed the death certificate (95% when it was the person's own doctor).

Five per cent of the doctors who were in the home after the death had been present at the time he died and 55% had come within an hour. Eighteen per cent had come between one and three hours later, 11% between three and six hours later, 9% later the same day and 2% on another day. Some of the dead persons were taken to hospital after the death, for example when worried relatives called an ambulance, and so the doctor did not come to the home. This sometimes led to confusion as to the place of death.[1]

> 'They'd taken him to hospital to see if they could bring him round but he was dead.'

Some doctors did not visit afterwards because they had seen the person a short while before he died. The relatives often had to collect the death certificate from his surgery. Two-thirds of the people who said a doctor did not visit after the death did not mind about this.[2]

> 'No need, it would have made no difference, he saw her the

[1] See Appendix IV: 'Comparison of data from interviews and death certificates'.

[2] Question 78(d): 'Would you have liked a doctor to come or not?'

same morning. When we rang another doctor was on duty. He said the doctor had seen her, hadn't he? He said, "Do you want me to come?" We said, "It's not necessary".'

'He came the day before so he just signed the death certificate—no need to come—I went for it.'

But the others would have liked the doctor to come and some were taken aback or alarmed when he did not.

'I thought they did—my sister had to go [to collect the death certificate]—I thought they'd come to certify the death in your own home. He said, "Come and get the certificate". I didn't like it.'

After death has been ascertained the body is washed and prepared. The undertaker was responsible for this in just over half the home deaths.[1] A relative helped with a quarter, friends and neighbours with nearly a fifth and a nurse with about a tenth. In about a twentieth of the home deaths the body was taken to a hospital, so no one at home was involved.

Women more often than men helped in caring for people before they died (two-thirds of the helpers were women). But men and women were equally involved in arrangements after death, and rather more of the men than women we interviewed negotiated with undertakers. (Forty-seven per cent of the men, 20% of the women, said they alone had been responsible for making arrangements with the undertaker.) This is consistent with other findings and theories on the male-female differentiation of family roles. Women tend to adopt 'expressive' roles, that is they are concerned principally with the maintenance of stability within the family, while men take on 'instrumental' roles concerned with maintaining the relationship of the family to the wider social order.[2]

Support of the bereaved

It has been recognised for a long time that grief as a result of bereavement can have pathogenic effects on the sufferers. The

[1] Question 76: 'Who washed and prepared ——'s body?'

[2] See Parsons, Talcott and Bates, Robert F., *Family Socialization and Interaction Process*, p. 23 and 47.

expression with which we are all familiar, 'broken heart', suggesting that people die of grief, and the acceptance of 'griefe' two centuries ago as a cause of death, are indicative of the widespread recognition of adverse reactions to bereavement. And outside the romantic sphere, in the scientific world, Lindemann in 1944 outlined his interpretation of the main features of acute grief which he considered to be a 'definite syndrome with psychological and somatic symptomatology'. This could be managed with psychiatric help where necessary, the psychiatrist sharing the patient's 'grief work'—'his efforts at extricating himself from the bondage to the deceased and at finding new patterns of rewarding interaction'.[1]

More recent studies of bereavement have reinforced the view that grief can be pathological and have called for preventive action from medical or psychiatric sources.[2] They have shown an increased mortality rate among widowers during the six months following the death of their wives,[3] and higher illness and medical consultation rates among widows in a similar period after their bereavement.[4] Another study showed a difference in mortality between the bereaved and a control group in the first year of bereavement,[5] and concluded that bereavement carried this increased risk, not just to widowed spouses, but in this case to other close relatives.

Non-professional people were the main source of support for the bereaved. Table 76 shows the people our respondents talked to and the kind of person they found most helpful. (Our respondents have been taken here as a sample of bereaved.)

The majority of the bereaved we interviewed said that relatives or close friends were the most appropriate people to talk to and the most helpful. One in ten felt they would not have liked to talk to anyone, and 13% found no one helpful. For some people, the interview was the first proper chance they had had to talk to anyone.

'You're the only person I've talked to about it. My relatives

[1] Lindemann, Erich, 'Symptomatology and management of acute grief'.

[2] Parkes, C. Murray, 'Grief as an illness'.

[3] Young, M., *et al.*, 'The mortality of widowers'.

[4] Parkes, C. Murray, 'Effects of bereavement on physical and mental health—a study of the medical records of widows'.

[5] Rees, W. Dewi and Lutkins, Sylvia G., 'Mortality of bereavement'.

TABLE 76 *The people respondents talked to and found most helpful since bereavement*

	Talked to[a]	*Most helpful*[b]
	%	%
Relative	63	63
Close friend	22	13
Outsider	5	3
Doctor	5	3
Clergyman	4	2
Nurse	1	1
Other person	2	2
No one	9	13
Number of respondents (=100%)[c]	718	

[a] Question 96: 'When someone close to you dies who do you feel it is best to talk to about how you feel?'
[b] Question 97: 'Who did you find most helpful?'
[c] This was not asked of those respondents who were not related to the person who died and who were not close friends.

never helped and I can't talk to them. I've never been close to any of them.'

'It's been a treat talking this afternoon—talked more than to anyone.'

But some could not bring themselves to discuss it with anyone.

'I can't talk to anyone. All my family have tried to help but they can't really.'

Some respondents thought that the relationship of the person they talked to was of secondary importance, the main point being that they wished to talk to someone who could understand and possibly share their grief.

'If you have relations they can probably understand your feelings—they probably share them.'

'My sister having gone through the same, she understands, and doesn't mind me going round any time.'

'Definitely a close friend of your choosing understands better than relatives.'

Bereavement is a time when religious faith might be a source of comfort and consolation. Of those 92% who said they belonged to a religious faith, two-thirds said they felt it had helped them at the time of the death,[1] three out of ten said it did not and the remainder were uncertain. Among those who said they belonged to the Church of England 62% said they found their faith helpful compared with 76% of the Roman Catholics and 79% of other Protestants.

A third of all the bereaved persons had been visited at home by a vicar, priest or minister since the death. Widows and daughters who used to live with the person who died were visited most, 41% and 47% respectively, while only a quarter of the widowers had been visited. However, more of the bereaved had been visited at home after the death by a member of the clergy than by any other professional, including their doctor. But we do not know whether they went to comfort the bereaved and offer help, or whether their visits were more concerned with funeral arrangements.

How much support and help do close relatives receive from general practitioners and other professional sources when they are bereaved? The people we interviewed who were most likely to be affected by the death were the widows and widowers, daughters and sons and other relatives, particularly those who had been living in the same household as the person who died.[2] The contact these people had with doctors since their bereavement is shown in Table 77.

Widows had the most contact with general practitioners. Seven out of ten had consulted their doctor since their bereavement compared with three-fifths of the widowers, half of them had done so in connection with their bereavement, compared with one-third of the widowers. Over a third of them had been visited at home by their own doctor compared with a sixth of

[1] Question 86: 'Have you a religious faith or belief which you feel helped you at the time of ——'s death?'

[2] Forty-two people are excluded from consideration in this section since they were not close friends or relatives of the deceased, and therefore were not asked about their 'bereavement'. Two of them lived in the same household as the person who died.

TABLE 77 *Contact of bereaved with medical practitioners*

	Relationship of respondent to person who died									
	Husband	*Wife*	*Daughter in same household*	*Female relative in same household*	*Daughter in other household*	*Other female relative in other household*	*Son*	*Other male relative*	*Close friend, etc.*[a]	*All respondents*[a]
Proportion who had consulted their general practitioner or other professional since bereavement[b]	59%	67%	49%	49%	44%	39%	30%	29%	41%	51%
Proportion consulting general practitioner, etc., in connection with bereavement[c]	32%	52%	35%	28%	30%	23%	8%	6%	23%	33%
Proportion who had been visited by own doctor since bereavement[d]	16%	37%	20%	36%	12%	10%	4%	9%	18%	21%
Proportion who had been prescribed something for shock, nerves, anxiety or sleeplessness[e]	23%	36%	20%	20%	18%	17%	3%	—	20%	22%
Number of respondents (=100%)	94	209	113	43	69	85	55	36	39	743

[a] These questions were not asked of the 42 respondents who were not relatives or close friends of the person who died.
[b] Question 92(a): 'Have you consulted a doctor, nurse or chemist professionally for yourself since —— died?'
[c] Question 92(c): 'Do you think it had anything to do with your bereavement or not?'
[d] Question 90: 'Have any of these people visited you at home since —— died?'
[e] Question 92(d): 'Did he give or sell you any tablets or medicine?' 'What were they for?'

the widowers. These differences suggest that there might be differences between men and women in the support over bereavement they seek and receive from general practitioners. In addition, daughters were much more likely than sons to have been visited by their doctors since their parent died, 17% against 4%; they were also more likely to have had a consultation in connection with their bereavement, 32% compared with 9%, and were more often given medicines for shock, nerves, anxiety or sleeplessness, 19% compared with 3%. (Women in general consult their doctors more often than men, but the differences here are greater than those usually observed.)[1] Gorer found similar differences between men and women mourners in his study.[2] Women may feel it more appropriate than men to seek support from general practitioners and others when they are bereaved. In addition general practitioners may feel it easier or more appropriate to offer support in such circumstances to women rather than men. Volkart and Michael argue that the role of male in Western society prohibits the expression of deep emotions, 'Thus in bereavement males may experience a conflict between their lifelong training in their sex role and the immediate situational demand for emotional expression as a bereaved person'.[3]

A less expected finding was that the proportion of respondents who had consulted a doctor since their bereavement decreased with their age, from 59% of those under 65 to 45% of those 75 or over. Likewise the proportions being prescribed medicines for shock, anxiety, sleeplessness or nerves decreased with age. If consultation reflects the extent to which people were disturbed by their bereavement it would seem that for older people death is not such an unusual and frightening experience as it is for younger people; they will have had more personal experience of people dying through the years, and will be more likely to have learned how to adjust to being bereaved. It may be, too, that they feel their bereavement is not for long; it will be curtailed by their own death.

Several writers have described a socialisation process in

[1] See, for example, Cartwright, Ann, *Patients and their Doctors*, p. 32, and Ashford, J. R. and Pearson, N. G., 'Who uses the health services and why?'

[2] Gorer, op. cit., pp. 53–4.

[3] Volkart, Edmund H. and Michael, Stanley T., 'Bereavement and mental health'.

prolonged terminal illness which gives rise to anticipatory bereavement before death. Lindemann[1] talks about 'anticipatory grief' and Gorer[2] of 'mourning before death'. Glaser and Strauss also discuss this.[3] The hypothesis is that relatives who have an opportunity to prepare themselves for bereavement may be better off after the death than those for whom the death was not expected. In this study there was some slight evidence that the more severely restricted the person who died had been and the longer the period of restriction before death the less likely were their relatives to seek medical care because of their bereavement. The proportion of relatives and close friends we interviewed who had consulted their general practitioners for some reason they associated with their bereavement declined from 72% when the person who died had not been restricted before the death to 60% when the person had been severely restricted for three months or longer, and the proportions taking medicines for shock, nerves, anxiety or sleeplessness from 60% to 35%.[4]

We asked the general practitioners in our study whether they thought that close bereaved should be given some medical or nursing supervision for a while.[5] Just over half (54%) thought not, almost a third (31%) that they should have some medical supervision and one in twelve that they should have some nursing supervision (this includes 3% who thought that they should have both medical and nursing supervision). One in ten gave qualified answers, and many more gave what appeared to be qualifying statements with their definite answer.

> 'Only if requested. Bereaved often wish to, and are better able to, deal with problems alone or with other relatives.'

> 'I always advise my patients that if I can help they know where to find me.'

> 'Not medical supervision. I visit in such circumstances to offer friendly sympathy.'

[1] Lindemann, op. cit. [2] Gorer, op. cit., p. 68.

[3] Glaser, Barney G. and Strauss, Anselm L., *Time for Dying*, pp. 56f.

[4] The first of these differences might have occurred by chance, the second was unlikely to have done so.

[5] Question 30: 'Do you think that close bereaved should be given some medical or nursing supervision for a while?'

These doctors said they thought the close bereaved should not receive medical or nursing supervision. Other doctors said 'no' quite definitely.

> 'Why? Death is a natural part of living.'

> 'Grief is best dealt with by family and friends.'

Some doctors had quite definite ideas about giving support.

> 'Six months. Much higher mortality rate for six months after for bereaved.'

> 'I visit for a fortnight or more.'

> 'Health visitor for one month. Ideally the health visitor should keep an eye on them.'

> 'Usually if elderly the district nurse or social worker continues to visit for a while.'

In practice, however, there were no differences in the proportions of close relatives who were visited at home by their doctors, district nurses or health visitors which could be related to the general practitioners' views on medical or nursing support for the bereaved. This suggests that doctors' views on this, or at any rate their replies to our questions, were unrelated to their actions.

One in five of the general practitioners thought that close bereaved should always be offered a sedative, half thought they should generally be offered one and a quarter said they should only exceptionally be offered one.[1] The remainder gave qualified answers. Once more, close relatives whose doctors said they should always be offered a sedative in such circumstances were no more likely to have been prescribed a medicine for shock, nerves, anxiety or sleeplessness than those whose doctor thought they should do so less often. All general practitioners were asked what they would prescribe for the close bereaved.[2] Forty-two per cent said that they would prescribe a drug acting as a sedative or tranquilliser, 8% a hypnotic, and 44% both sedative and hypnotic. Only 4% said they would prescribe an

[1] Question 28: 'Do you think that close bereaved should: always be offered a sedative, generally be offered a sedative, only exceptionally be offered a sedative?'

[2] Question 29: 'What do you prescribe in such circumstances?'

antidepressant, and 20% of the drugs mentioned had other functions in addition. Over half of the drugs mentioned, 57%, contained a barbiturate.[1]

The district nurses and health visitors in the study were also asked if they thought that the bereaved should be given medical or nursing supervision. Three-quarters thought they should, one in eight thought not and one in ten gave a qualified answer. The views of the doctors, district nurses and health visitors are shown in Table 78.

TABLE 78 *Professionals' views on type of support for the bereaved*[a]

	General practitioner	*District nurse*	*Health visitor*
	%	%	%
Medical supervision	28	35	39
Nursing supervision	5	24	19
Both medical and nursing supervision	3	17	26
Neither of these	54	14	5
Qualified answer	10	10	11
Number of respondents (=100%)	320	502	75

[a] Question 30 (doctors), 21 (nurses): 'Do you think that close bereaved should be given some medical or nursing supervision for a while?'

Health visitors and district nurses were more likely than doctors to think the bereaved should be given medical or nursing or both kinds of supervision. Most of the doctors who said that the bereaved should receive some supervision said that they themselves should provide it. Fifty-two per cent of all the district nurses and 65% of the health visitors said that the bereaved should receive medical attention. Some were obviously influenced by their own experience of bereavement—8% of the nurses and health visitors were themselves widowed, separated or divorced.

[1] All the general practitioners were asked this question. Less of those who said that the close bereaved should only exceptionally be offered a sedative, 77%, said what kind of drug they would prescribe, than those who said they should always be offered a sedative, 93%.

'Something you have to go through yourself to understand.'

'Should be given help—seen by doctor. I wasn't and collapsed. Should be examined by doctor a fortnight afterwards.'

It was often thought that if the district nurse or health visitor was attending the bereaved periodically, she could refer them to their doctor should the need arise.

'Depends on them. Could tell G.P. if you thought they needed anything else.' (This nurse said they should receive nursing supervision.)

Health visitors and district nurses were asked who they thought was the most appropriate person to provide nursing support for the bereaved.[1] Not surprisingly more of the health visitors than district nurses thought that health visitors were the more appropriate and vice versa. In fact, half of each group thought that they were the more appropriate source of support for the bereaved. Only 7% of the health visitors thought that district nurses alone were appropriate and 42% thought the responsibility should be shared. A third of the nurses thought the health visitor alone should be responsible for this and one in six thought they should have joint responsibility or gave qualified answers.

'The one who has had most to do with them because that's the person they know best' (district nurse).

'If the district nurse has been involved in nursing patient she would know the family and could do it best. If the district nurse hasn't been involved then the health visitor should provide support' (health visitor).

One reason often given in favour of the health visitor providing the support was that she would have more time to visit where actual nursing care was not needed. The most frequent counter-

[1] Question 22: 'In our pilot study opinions of health visitors and district nurses were divided about who should provide nursing supervision or support for the bereaved. Do you think the most appropriate person is the health visitor or the district nurse?'

argument was that the district nurse would know the family better.

> 'They [health visitors] have more time—we get someone on the books as soon as we lose one' (district nurse).

> 'A district nurse is already known to the family' (district nurse).

The nurses and health visitors who were involved in the care of people in our sample were asked about their contact with the bereaved. Only 15% of all the nurses and health visitors said they had some professional contact with the bereaved, most commonly the widowed spouse, and about half of these had been in contact with the bereaved person for over a month.[1] For the most part, however, their involvement ceased with, or soon after, the death of their patient.

Few of the bereaved said they would have liked a visit from a doctor, nurse or other professional if they had not had one. Five per cent would have appreciated a visit from a doctor, 3% from a vicar, priest or minister, 1% from a district nurse. So although a number of the professionals felt they had a part to play in the support of bereaved relatives the people themselves turned more to their families and friends.

Adaptation and adjustment

Bereaved people have to adjust to their new state while they are preoccupied with a painful struggle to master their grief. Marris writes about the adaptation of widows:

> 'For months, even years after his death, her energies may be so absorbed in this struggle, and her feelings so deeply disturbed as to affect all her needs and her response to those who try to meet them.'[2]

Our interviewers often reported people breaking down and crying during the interview. Sometimes the interview had to be discontinued, or was refused altogether because the respondent, who was not necessarily the widow or widower, was too

[1] Question 34: 'Did you visit ——'s home after the death at all?' Question 35: 'Why did you visit then?'

[2] Marris, Peter, *Widows and their families*, p. 10.

upset. These emotional reactions sometimes occurred among those interviewed nine months after the person died. One study showed evidence of social disengagement in widows and widowers three years after their bereavement.[1] For some people the process of adjustment is a long and painful business.

The death of a close relative may also mean material changes in people's way of life. We asked the relatives and close friends we interviewed if they had made any changes and if they were planning any changes in their way of living since the death.[2]

TABLE 79 *Changes made and planned by respondents*

	Changes made	*Changes planned*
Type of change	%	%
None	71	81
Household composition	8	13
Household arrangements	4	2
Work	9	3
Other	11	2
Number of respondents (=100%)[a]	721	706

[a] Percentages add to more than 100 as some respondents made or planned more than one type of change.

Seventy-one per cent said they had made no changes and four-fifths of these said they were not planning any. The changes which they said they had made, or intended to make, are shown in Table 79. The most common one which they said they had made was in their work, 9%, and the most common one they planned was in the composition of their household, that is, they were mostly going to move either to a new house or to live with someone else.

However, it seemed that there were other far-reaching consequences of the death that the respondents did not mention or possibly would not admit. The fact that they said they had

[1] Parkes, C. Murray, and Brown, R. J., 'Health after bereavement'.

[2] Question 93: 'Have you made any changes in your way of living since —— died?' Question 94: 'Are you planning any (other) changes?'

made no changes meant that they had done nothing to accommodate for the one great change which had occurred—the loss of one of their relatives or close friends, and the subsequent effects that this loss had. Not only did the death bring an end to what in most cases was an important personal relationship, but it also entailed, in some cases, the loss of the major source of income to the household. The death of a husband or wife involves the breaking-up of a team. A widower might never have done any housework; a widow might find herself excluded from social events. For some the death meant a release from the hard work of looking after an incapacitated and invalid relative.

Ninety-one per cent of the husbands or wives who used to live only with the spouse who died were living alone at the time of the interview. Widowers were more likely than widows to be living alone, 63% compared with 49%. More of the widows than the widowers were living with other relatives, usually sons or daughters, 46% and 29% respectively. These findings are rather surprising as other data suggest that widows are more likely to live alone than widowers.[1] Widows may be more likely than widowers to have to give up their home because they can no longer afford its upkeep.

Twenty-nine per cent of the respondents admitted to having some particular worry or anxiety since the death.[2] Financial worries were those most frequently reported—by 14%. Ten per cent had legal difficulties with the will, 7% had problems with their house or tenancy and a further 8% reported a variety of other problems. For example one man, seen three months after his wife's death, was so upset that he had still not been able to face up to the necessary arrangements with his bank and for his house.

> 'The bank kept asking me to go—we had a joint account—not short of money, but must change it. My wife didn't make a will, the house was in both our names so I must do

[1] General Register Office, *Sample Census 1966. Household Composition Tables*, p. 315.

[2] Question 95: 'Since —— died have you had any particular worries or anxieties such as: financial worries, legal ones—to do with the will, problems with the house or tenancy, anything else?'

> something about that. Everything is in a mess, all my fault. I can't face doing anything about it.'

A third of those who had worries about something did not consult anyone about them. When they did consult people, two-thirds felt they had got some help.

In his study of widows Marris tells how difficult it was for some to adapt.[1] They frequently felt their dead husband was present. They found old routines were difficult to break, and at the same time provoked distressing memories. Some found it difficult to accept the fact of their bereavement. Some of these phenomena were reported in our study. Feelings of loneliness were frequently mentioned. This seems an inevitable consequence of the death of a close relative or friend.

In conclusion

In the preceding description of death and bereavement based on data from our study we have not discussed some of the more interesting ideas of other researchers. This is because the limited information we have does not support their hypotheses but we feel this may be a reflection of the superficiality of this part of our data.

Parkes has suggested:

> 'Therapy should, when possible, start before the bereavement and it is not uncommon for a person to get over the worst of his grief before the actual death has occurred. It is important for doctors and relatives of a seriously ill person to see that those most concerned are aware of his approaching death. Too often the true prognosis is kept dark with the object of sparing the feelings of the closest relatives, as a result of which death when it comes is not expected and the shock is great.'[2]

Our study did not show a difference between relatives who knew that the person was dying and those who did not in the only measures we have of their possible distress—consultation with a doctor and being given medicine for such symptoms as anxiety, shock, nerves or sleeplessness. We did find, however,

[1] Marris, op. cit., pp. 10–30.

[2] Parkes, C. Murray, 'Grief as an illness'.

that the longer and more severe the restrictions suffered by the person who died the less likely were their relatives to be taking medicines for symptoms possibly associated with distress and bereavement.

There are many factors complicating attempts to relate knowledge and behaviour before death to measures of distress. Older people who may be more practised at managing their grief did not consult their doctor as much as younger bereaved people. Husbands and wives were less likely to know that someone was dying than sons, daughters and other relatives. Women seemed to be more expressive than men about their difficulties in adjusting to bereavement.

Then there is the possibility that seeking professional help in bereavement may be an indication that the bereaved person is not denying his grief. Although relatives and friends were the main source of support for the bereaved, Gorer has described how reactions to mourning as if it were 'a weakness, a self-indulgence, a reprehensible bad habit instead of a psychological necessity' make some bereaved feel that they must mourn in private and hide their grief from family and friends.[1] If this happens, those who do not seek professional help may well be more in need of it than those who consult their doctor.

[1] Gorer, op. cit., p. 113.

11

SOCIAL CLASS AND AREA VARIATIONS

In this penultimate chapter the twelve study areas are described and variations between them in the care given to the dying are analysed. Variations in the care given to people in different social classes are then examined.

The twelve study areas

The populations of the twelve study areas and the administrative districts they covered are shown in Appendix I. Table 80 gives some basic statistics about them. They have been divided into four groups.

The relatively well-off urban areas were Cheshire North-East, Hillingdon, Brentwood and Eastbourne. *Cheshire North-East* is the most prosperous of the twelve areas with the highest proportion of household amenities, cars, and professional workers, and the lowest rate of overcrowding. It is the only one of the four areas in the relatively well-off group that is in the north. *Hillingdon* is a relatively well-off borough to the west of London. *Brentwood* registration district in Essex is made up of the two urban districts of Brentwood and Basildon. Both Hillingdon and Brentwood have comparatively good amenities and a high proportion of cars. The other area in this group, *Eastbourne,* is rather different. It has a high proportion of old people aged 65 or more, 28% compared with 12% in England and Wales. Associated with this it has a comparatively low average household size (2·5 persons compared with 3·0 in England and Wales) and this probably accounts for a low proportion of household amenities compared with other areas in this group. But like them it has a higher than average proportion of men in professional occupations. Cheshire, Brentwood and Eastbourne increased their populations by 10% or

TABLE 80 *Statistics for twelve study areas*

	Relatively well-off urban areas				*Partly rural areas in the south*		*More rural areas in the north*		*Less well-off urban areas*				
	Cheshire North East	*Hillingdon*	*Brentwood and Basildon*	*Eastbourne*	*Isle of Wight*	*Thanet*	*Northumberland North Second*	*Bridgend*	*Barking*	*Birmingham*	*Teesside South*	*St Helens*	*England and Wales*
Proportion of population in rural districts in 1969	3%	—	—	—	20%	18%	57%	60%	—	—	6%[c]	—	21%
Birth wastage rates 1969[a]	25	30	23	28	27	25	25	36	32	34	34[d]	38	31
Census 1966													
Proportion of households with exclusive use of various amenities[b]	93%	91%	89%	77%	76%	79%	79%	71%	81%	64%	69%[e]	62%	72%
Proportion of people in households:													
With a car	69%	66%	66%	42%	52%	47%	53%	53%	47%	44%	41%[e]	33%	51%
With density over 1 person per room	5%	8%	10%	6%	7%	8%	17%	9%	12%	18%	15%[e]	15%	11%
Proportion of economically active or retired males in:													
Professional occupations	11%	7%	6%	5%	4%	4%	3%	3%	2%	3%	4%[e]	2%	4%
Unskilled occupations	4%	6%	6%	7%	7%	7%	8%	8%	12%	9%	13%[e]	17%	8%
Proportion of population aged 65 or more	10%	10%	9%	28%	19%	21%	14%	11%	11%	11%	10%[e]	12%	12%
Migration balance in 5 years per 1,000 resident population	144	9	100	100	68	88	−33	47	−66	−54	4[e]	−67	

[a] Number of stillbirths and deaths under 1 year per 1,000 live and still births.
[b] Hot water tap, inside water closet and fixed bath.
[c] Based on figures for 1967. The areas for 1969 had changed.
[d] The figure relates to Teesside C.B. which covers a population 42% greater than the registration district.
[e] Census data omits Guisborough U.D. (part) and Saltburn & Marske-by-the-Sea (part) which contain 0·5% of the population of the registration district. The whole of Stokesley R.D. is included although only 50% of that area is in the registration district.

more between 1961 and 1966. Hillingdon's population size remained relatively stationary. Brentwood and Cheshire had low birth wastage rates.[1]

Partly rural areas are Thanet and the Isle of Wight both in the south and with just under a fifth of their populations in rural districts. The other outstanding feature of these areas is that about a fifth of their population is aged 65 or more—presumably their coast-lines and seaside towns attract people from other areas when they retire. Both had expanding populations.

More rural areas were Northumberland North Second and Bridgend in South Wales where over half the population lived in rural districts. Both are north of the Bristol-Wash line. The main differences between them are that Bridgend had an expanding, Northumberland a contracting, population; Bridgend a high birth wastage rate, Northumberland a low one.

The less-well-off urban areas were Barking, Birmingham, Teesside South and St Helens—the first south and the other three north of the Bristol-Wash line. Barking is on the east side of London, Birmingham is the largest county borough in the country, Teesside South covers the area of Teesside C.B. on the south of the Tees, and St Helens is in Lancashire. All these areas have relatively crowded households and few people in professional occupations. All except Barking have lower than average household amenities and higher than average birth wastage rates. The populations of Barking, Birmingham and St Helens declined by 5% or more in the five years before the 1966 Census. In Teesside South emigration and immigration were almost equally balanced.

Our survey data on the occupations and amenities of the people who died in the areas reflect a similar picture (see Table 81). In Cheshire, Hillingdon and Brentwood relatively high proportions of the people who died had been in non-manual occupations and lived in households with telephones. In Cheshire and Hillingdon a high proportion also lived in households with cars. Eastbourne had an even higher proportion of people in non-manual occupations (presumably because it is the well-off who can afford to retire there), a high proportion of households with telephones but a low proportion of households

[1] Number of stillbirths and deaths under one year per 1,000 live and stillbirths.

TABLE 81 *Survey data for study areas*

	Relatively well-off urban areas				*Partly rural areas in the south*		*More rural areas in the north*		*Less well-off urban areas*				
	Cheshire North East	*Hillingdon*	*Brentwood and Basildon*	*Eastbourne*	*Isle of Wight*	*Thanet*	*Northumberland North Second*	*Bridgend*	*Barking*	*Birmingham*	*Teesside South*	*St Helens*	*All areas*
Proportion of people who died:													
Who had worked in non-manual occupations[a]	46%	45%	41%	66%	40%	32%	27%	20%	13%	28%	18%	14%	32%
Who lived in households:													
With a car[b]	51%	55%	30%	35%	51%	20%	47%	43%	30%	37%	17%	25%	36%
With a telephone[b]	51%	48%	44%	50%	51%	26%	30%	24%	24%	39%	25%	13%	35%
With own inside W.C.[c]	80%	92%	84%	78%	80%	82%	87%	65%	93%	70%	59%	67%	78%
Who had lived in the same house for 20 years or more[c]	31%	53%	30%	28%	26%	35%	42%	48%	57%	48%	41%	58%	41%

[a] Based on data for complete sample from death certificates.
[b] Excluding those under 65 who died unexpectedly, and those who had been in a hospital or institution for 12 months or more before they died.
[c] Excluding those under 65 who died unexpectedly.

with cars. People may attach more importance to telephones than cars when they retire and some may stop driving as they get older.

Of the four rural or partly rural areas, the Isle of Wight had the highest proportion of people in non-manual occupations and of people in households with telephones. Only two-thirds of the households in Bridgend had their own inside lavatory.

Other differences of note were that St Helens had a high proportion of Roman Catholics—36% of the respondents there said they were Catholics, compared with 9% in the rest of the sample—whereas Bridgend had a high proportion of non-conformists and other Protestants (apart from Church of England): 50% compared with 14% in the other areas taken together.

Area variations in care

Area variations in place of death and in household composition for the people in our survey are shown in Table 82. The proportion of home deaths was higher in the north than in the south, 45% against 35%. The proportion of people who had been in hospitals or other institutions for a year or more before their death was relatively high, 17%, in the three areas—Eastbourne, the Isle of Wight and Thanet—with a particularly high proportion of old people aged 65 or more, but it was also high in Brentwood, 21%, compared with 5% in the other areas taken together. The proportion of people who lived with younger relatives was lower in the south than in the north, 32% compared with 47%, and within the south it was relatively low in the three areas with a high proportion of old people—24% compared with 39% in the other three southern areas combined.

Help received from various official sources and from friends and relatives is shown for the twelve study areas in Table 83. Rather more people in the north than in the south had been helped by a district nurse: 40% compared with 32%. Conversely other nurses, who were often private ones, had more often been involved in the care of people dying in the south than in the north: 7% against 4%. (The proportion was particularly high in Eastbourne, 21%.) Related to this, other nurses more often helped people dying in the relatively well-off urban areas than in other types of area: 11% against 3%.

TABLE 82 *Area variations in place of death and previous household composition*

	Relatively well-off urban areas				*Partly rural areas in the south*		*More rural areas in the north*		*Less well-off urban areas*			
	Cheshire North-East	*Hillingdon*	*Brentwood and Basildon*	*Eastbourne*	*Isle of Wight*	*Thanet*	*Northumberland North Second*	*Bridgend*	*Barking*	*Birmingham*	*Teesside South*	*St Helens*
Place of death from death certificate	%	%	%	%	%	%	%	%	%	%	%	%
In general hospitals	35	50	45	46	51	44	37	31	54	45	50	36
In other institutions	4	9	20	19	9	12	10	5	5	11	6	15
In own home	55	39	31	33	35	43	48	56	29	33	38	39
Elsewhere	6	2	4	2	5	1	5	8	12	11	6	10
Number of deaths (=100%)	80	80	80	80	80	80	80	80	80	80	80	80
Household composition	%	%	%	%	%	%	%	%	%	%	%	%
In institution all year	—	3	21	19	16	15	6	6	7	6	6	6
On own	17	10	12	8	10	14	20	8	15	9	20	9
With spouse only	29	35	18	35	26	37	21	23	40	32	21	27
With relatives of a younger generation	43	50	36	13	35	25	39	54	32	47	50	49
Other	11	2	13	25	13	9	14	9	6	6	3	9
Number of deaths (=100%)	65	58	67	63	62	59	70	65	72	68	70	66

TABLE 83 *Area variations in help received from various officials and from relatives and friends*

	Relatively well-off urban areas				*Partly rural areas in the south*		*More rural areas in the north*		*Less well-off urban areas*			
	Cheshire North East	*Hillingdon*	*Brentwood and Basildon*	*Eastbourne*	*Isle of Wight*	*Thanet*	*Northumberland North Second*	*Bridgend*	*Barking*	*Birmingham*	*Teesside South*	*St Helens*
Help given by:	%	%	%	%	%	%	%	%	%	%	%	%
District nurse	52	27	31	33	44	25	53	33	28	38	33	31
Health visitor	—	4	6	19	8	—	10	4	6	7	25	9
Other nurse	7	4	14	21	—	6	3	6	—	3	3	—
Home help	18	4	18	6	8	4	10	10	13	12	18	7
Special laundry services	—	—	2	2	—	—	—	—	4	7	—	2
Chiropodist	12	8	16	19	6	19	15	10	2	9	16	11
Clergy	30	17	29	23	36	17	56	49	11	21	25	58
Other	10	15	12	15	6	6	10	10	13	19	18	16
No official	18	50	41	42	40	50	23	29	49	38	28	29
Average number of friends/relatives helping	3·4	2·4	2·5	2·1	1·9	1·9	3·2	3·4	2·6	2·9	3·4	2·7
Number of deaths excluding those in hospital or institution and unexpected deaths of people under 65 (=100%)	60	52	51	50	50	48	62	52	54	60	61	55

In the areas with a high proportion of elderly people the people who died were less likely to have had a home help: 6% compared with 12% in other areas. Apart from these differences there did not appear to be any particular pattern in the proportions receiving help from a district nurse or other local authority service. For example, the proportions did not differ significantly in urban or rural areas, or between the urban areas that were well-off or less well-off. Clergy were more likely to have helped in the north than in the south, 39% against 22%, and in rural or partly rural areas than in urban areas, 41% against 27%.

But there were wide variations in the proportion helped by a health visitor, from over a fifth in Eastbourne and Teesside to none at all in some areas. Presumably this reflects the local authority's policy in the sort of work allocated to health visitors, or the number of health visitors available.

The average number of friends and relatives who helped was low, 1·9, for the three areas with a high proportion of old people—Eastbourne, the Isle of Wight and Thanet. It was higher, 2·5, for other southern areas and higher still, 3·2, for areas in the north.

So far we have just been considering differences between the north and south, between urban and rural areas, between areas with high proportions of elderly people and the rest and between the relatively well-off and not so well-off areas. But how do the different indices we have considered relate to each other for our twelve study areas? This is shown in Table 84 which indicates which pairs of indices appear to be associated, either positively or negatively. The indices considered were (1) the proportion of deaths in peoples' own homes, (2) the proportion of long-term institutional deaths, (3) the proportion living with relatives of a younger generation, (4) the proportion helped by a district nurse, (5) the proportion helped by a health visitor, (6) the average number of friends and relatives who helped, (7) the proportion of the population aged 65 or more, (8) the birth wastage rate and (9) the proportion of economically active or retired males in professional occupations.[1]

[1] The number of hospital beds in the region per head of the population was not related to the proportion dying at home, the proportion of long-term

TABLE 84 *Relationship between various indices in the twelve study areas*

	Correlation coefficients								
	1	2	3	4	5	6	7	8	9
1. The proportion of deaths in peoples' own homes	—								
2. The proportion of long-term institutional deaths	*d*	—							
3. The proportion living with relatives of a younger generation before they died or went into hospital	0·39	*d*	—						
4. The proportion helped by a district nurse	0·45	−0·29	0·10	—					
5. The proportion helped by a health visitor	−0·35	0·17	−0·11	−0·03	—				
6. The average number of relatives and friends who helped	0·55	−0·70[b]	0·69[b]	0·42	0·12	—			
7. The proportion of the population aged 65 or more	−0·17	0·60[a]	−0·83[c]	−0·06	0·23	−0·65[a]	—		
8. The birth wastage rate	−0·02	−0·45	0·56	−0·34	0·27	0·34	−0·29	—	
9. The proportion of economically active or retired males in professional occupations	0·34	−0·16	−0·01	0·32	−0·28	0·11	−0·12	−0·54	—

[a] $0{\cdot}02 \leqslant p < 0{\cdot}05$ [b] $0{\cdot}01 < p \leqslant 0{\cdot}02$ [c] $p \leqslant 0{\cdot}001$

[d] It is inappropriate to calculate these because the two indices are mutually exclusive, and there is therefore a built-in association between the two.

A high proportion of elderly people in an area usually went with a high proportion of long-term institutional or hospital deaths, a low proportion of people who lived with relatives of a younger generation and a low average number of friends and relatives helping with care. A high number of relatives and friends who helped was associated with a low proportion of long-term institutional deaths and a high proportion of people living with relatives of a younger generation.

The proportion of deaths in people's own homes, and the proportions helped by a district nurse or health visitor, were not correlated with any of the other indices. If the proportion dying at home is taken as an index of need for home nursing care in an area, these findings suggest that the services in an area were not related to the needs of that area. Nor was there any apparent statistical relationship between the help given by district nurses and health visitors on an area basis.[1]

Movement to a seaside area on retirement might appear to isolate people from younger relatives and to mean that people are more likely to spend the last year of their lives in a hospital or institution. But an alternative explanation is that people who move on retirement are those with no close friends or relatives living near them. The proportion of people who died who had any living children was comparatively low, 55%, in Eastbourne compared with between 71% and 93% in the other areas and 78% altogether. It was not particularly low in the other two 'retirement areas': 74% in Thanet, 80% in the Isle of Wight.

Social class

Death in many respects appeared to be the equaliser it is so often reputed to be. We found no social class differences in reported symptoms or restrictions or the type of help people needed except that working-class people more often needed financial help: 26% compared with 14% of the middle-class people who died. The only difference in their place of death was in the proportions dying in private nursing homes; this

institutional deaths, or the proportion of the population aged 65 and over in the study areas.

[1] See also Davies, Bleddyn P., *et al., Variations in Services for the Aged*, p. 13, and Moseley, L. G., 'Variations in socio-medical services for the aged'.

fell from 6% in Social Class I, the professional group, to 1% in Social Classes IV and V, the semi-skilled and unskilled group.

Another study of deaths[1] (excluding those from malignant neoplasms, fatal accidents and sudden deaths from coronary heart disease and confined to deaths of people aged from 15 to 74) suggested that fewer of the patients in Social Classes IV and V had been referred to hospital than of those in I, II or III. We did not find any difference in the proportions who had been in contact with hospitals as in-patients or out-patients in the last year of their lives. Taking the proportions who died in general N.H.S. hospitals there is a slight trend in the opposite direction. Excluding deaths from cancer, and accidents and unexpected deaths of people under 65 from heart conditions, the proportions dying in a general hospital rose from 34% of those in Social Classes I and II to 51% of those in Social Class V.

There were, of course, clear variations in housing conditions and household equipment with social class. These are shown in Table 85.

The gradient was most marked for the telephone and an unshared indoor W.C. and least definite for a washing machine. It is clear that middle-class houses were more likely to have the amenities and equipment which make it easier to care for people who are ill at home.

The proportion who regarded the deceased person's house or flat as very convenient for them declined from 73% in Social Classes I and II to 47% in Social Class V. There were no class differences in the proportion living alone, with just a spouse or with people of a younger generation. Neither did the proportion visited by a district nurse, health visitor, home help, vicar or priest vary with the person's social class. But more of the middle-class than of the working-class people who died had been helped by a chiropodist, 15% against 8%, and by 'another' nurse,[2] 9% compared with 3%.

There were no class differences in the number of general practitioner consultations, home visits or night calls, nor in

[1] Alderson, M. R., 'Referral to hospital among a representative sample of adults who died'.

[2] That is a nurse who was not thought, by the respondent, to be a district nurse or health visitor. Most of these were private nurses but some male district nurses may also have been included.

TABLE 85 *Variations in housing and household equipment with social classes*

	I	II	III Skilled		IV	V	
	Profes-sional	*Inter-mediate*	*Non-manual*	*Manual*	*Semi-skilled*	*Unskilled*	*All Classes*
Proportion in household with:							
Own bathroom with running hot and cold water	92%	90%	82%	81%	71%	68%	79%
Own indoor W.C.	96%	94%	86%	77%	70%	60%	78%
Washing machine	58%	66%	55%	57%	59%	39%	56%
Spin dryer	63%	59%	42%	45%	42%	25%	44%
Car	63%	58%	34%	37%	24%	20%	36%
Telephone	83%	63%	38%	30%	19%	10%	35%
Proportion of people who died who had no stairs or steps between bedroom and W.C.	79%	80%	66%	63%	62%	65%	67%
Number of deaths (=100%)[a]	24	97	76	217	152	65	655

[a] Excluding those who had been in hospital or institution for a year or more before they died and those under 65 who died unexpectedly. Small numbers for whom inadequate information was available have also been excluded when calculating percentages.

respondents' views about whether the person's doctor was easy to talk to or had time to discuss things. Comparison of the general practitioners of working- and middle-class people revealed no differences in the number of patients they looked after, their access to hospital beds, the proportion in group practice, the proportion with any local health authority staff attached to them, or in their views. But there was a clear trend in the proportion of people who died who had a domiciliary visit by a consultant—from 29% of those in the professional group to 6% in the unskilled.

Although working-class people are likely to have greater needs because of the more difficult conditions under which they are living, help from official sources and other agencies did not seem to counterbalance this.

There was no appreciable difference between middle- and working-class people in the average numbers of relatives, friends and neighbours who had helped to look after them, but the types of people involved were different. Working-class people were more often helped by daughters and sons, middle-class people by friends and neighbours.[1] This can be seen from Table 86. The average number of daughters who helped was 0·40 for middle-class people who died, 0·62 for working class.

The difference in the proportion receiving help from daughters and sons seems to be explained by the existence of living children; 68% of the middle-class and 83% of the working-class had one living child or more and the average number of children was 1·35 for the middle-class, 2·20 for the working class. There was no difference between the classes in the proportion with children whom they had not seen in the year before they died.

A comparison of the proximity of relatives who helped but did not live in the same household did not reveal any class differences, but the friends and neighbours who helped lived nearer to the working-class people who died. This is shown in Table 87. It suggests that middle-class people drew on a more scattered circle of friends to compensate for their fewer rela-

[1] This is in line with differences found on other studies, that middle-class people rely more on friends for social contacts, working-class on relatives. See Willmott, Peter, and Young, Michael, *Family and Class in a London Suburb*, p. 110.

TABLE 86 *The relatives and friends who helped*

	Middle-class people who died		*Working-class people who died*	
	%		%	
Husband or wife	16		16	
Daughter	14	23	21	35
Son	9		14	
Daughter-in-law	3	6	5	10
Son-in-law	3		5	
Other relative	23		21	
Friend or neighbour	28		17	
Other person	4		1	
Number of helpers (=100%)	509		1,246	

TABLE 87 *The proximity of friends and neighbours who helped*

	Middle-class people who died	*Working-class people who died*
	%	%
Within 10 minutes' walk	66	92
Within half-hour journey	25	5
Half hour but less than 1 hour	6	2
1 hour but less than 2 hours	1	1
2 hours or more	2	—
Number of friends and neighbours who helped but did not live in same household (=100%)	124	193

tives.[1] The friends or neighbours who helped the working-class people were more often neighbours.

Conclusions

Data from this survey do not obviously reinforce either

[1] See also Bott, Elizabeth, *Family and Social Network*, p. 122.

Titmuss's argument that the middle class make more effective use of health services[1] or Rein's refutation of the argument and his claim that the health service is equitable.[2] Both could select some parts of the information to support their theses.

Apart from the greater use by the middle class of domiciliary consultation, chiropody services and other nurses there was no evidence of class differences in the extent to which they used N.H.S. hospital services, general practitioners or various local authority services. And the limited data we have about needs in terms of reported symptoms, restrictions and perceived needs for care suggest that there were no major class differences in these, except for a greater need for financial help among the working class.

Although the working class had more relatives, and particularly children, to help them, the middle class depended on their friends to a greater extent, so that each had similar numbers of people to help them. The main discrepancy in their ability to cope with illness at home arose from the poorer housing conditions and fewer amenities of the working class. The services did not counterbalance this disadvantage.

The differences in services between areas seemed unrelated to likely needs. The National Health Service may mean that care is no longer clearly related inversely to need.[3] But there is little or no evidence of any positive correlation between the two. Our study supports the conclusions of an earlier one that:

'1. The large variations in the services for the aged do not coincide with variations in need.

2. If an area is poorly provided with one service it is not likely that this will be compensated for by high provision in some complementary service.'[4]

[1] Titmuss, Richard M., *Commitment to Welfare* and *Essays on The Welfare State.*

[2] Rein, Martin, 'Social class and the utilisation of medical care services' and 'Social class and the health service'.

[3] Hart, Julian Tudor, 'The inverse care law'.

[4] Moseley, op. cit.

12

SUMMARY AND CONCLUSIONS

There are a number of gaps in this picture of the last year of people's lives. The most important one is that we do not know what the people themselves thought about the care they received, about dying at home or in hospital, or about knowing or not knowing that they were dying. Another omission is that we were unable to include 18% of the people from our random sample. Some people who were isolated, with few relatives or friends to care for them or take an interest when they were admitted to a hospital or institution, have probably been omitted from the study, simply because there was no one who could tell us about their last year. A further drawback is that we probably attempted too much. In trying to describe people's needs and the care they were given by relatives and friends, hospitals, general practitioners, district nurses, home helps and others we collected a mass of statistics as well as detailed descriptions of individual circumstances. The danger is that our more important findings have been buried in a welter of detail. In this final chapter we try to put our results into perspective and to highlight some of the ways in which services could be improved. The study has certainly revealed many inadequacies in present services.

Inadequate level of services

Analysis of who dies in hospital and information from general practitioners suggest that there are insufficient hospital beds or beds in appropriate homes for some groups of patients. The shortage seems particularly acute for old people needing long-term nursing care,[1] and it is these people who need a great deal of care from community services if they cannot be looked after in hospitals or institutions.

[1] See also Butler, John R. and Pearson, Mary, *Who goes home?*, p. 63.

But the resources of the community services for this sort of care are also often inadequate. Nearly two-thirds of the district nurses felt they would like to give more time to patients with a terminal illness. The way they had to hurry from one patient to another meant that the nurses often could not talk to patients and give them and their relatives the help and support they would like to, nor could many of them give their patients all the nursing care they felt was appropriate.

Home help services, too, were often deficient. Not only could more than twice as many of the people who died have done with a home help, but almost half of those who had such help were thought by their relatives or friends to have needed it more often. There were also difficulties about mobilising help quickly in a crisis. This study, and others,[1] also revealed the need for a rather different service—someone between a district nurse and a home help. Bathing services and help at night were needed more often, and so were services for helping with the care of incontinent people at home.

Another service which was often unsatisfactory for the care of the elderly and sick at home was housing. Almost a quarter of the people aged 65 or more who died had an outside lavatory. Washing machines, spin dryers and telephones would often have been helpful in relieving the heavy burden of care. Telephones facilitate contact between elderly or infirm people and their relatives and friends. They also enable people to get in touch with services in a crisis.

All these—more services, better housing and the provision of equipment—require money. Central and local government need to be persuaded that investment in them is worthwhile. The pay-off is death with greater dignity.

Co-ordination of services

Not only more services, better services and sometimes rather different sorts of services are needed. We also need to ensure better co-ordination between services, so that people get help from the most appropriate source and so that there is no danger of falling through a gap where no one accepts responsibility for

[1] See Warren, M. D., *et al.*, 'Problems of emergency admissions to London hospitals', and Hockey, Lisbeth, *Feeling the Pulse*.

care. Various possible loopholes have been highlighted by this study:

Patient – general practitioner One of the most disconcerting findings was the high proportion of symptoms for which apparently no one had been consulted. Over half of those suffering from an unpleasant smell and of those with loss of bladder but not bowel control were said not to have sought help from any professional person about it. This proportion was two-fifths for those with depression and a quarter of those with loss of bowel control. Most of the people with these symptoms had seen their general practitioner since the symptom developed but apparently had not asked him about it either because of embarrassment or fear or because they felt he could do nothing to help. Possibly they had more pressing things they wanted to ask him about and felt they must limit their queries and not bother the doctor with all their problems. Certainly other studies have also shown that the amount of unmet need for care from general practitioners is high among old people.[1] If elderly patients are reluctant or hesitant to bring symptoms to their doctor's notice, this reinforces the argument for check-ups and investigations initiated by the doctor.

General practitioner – hospital Many general practitioners find difficulty in arranging admission to an appropriate N.H.S. institution for various groups of patients. If they experience such difficulties frequently it may discourage them from attempting to arrange it for other patients and less suitable alternatives will be sought. Most doctors felt the difficulties arose because there were not enough beds available, particularly chronic hospital and geriatric beds. But, one in seven felt that there was inadequate consultation between them and the hospital medical staff about the admission of patients, and the greater their difficulty in obtaining admission the more often they asked for domiciliary consultations.

Even when general practitioners are satisfied with the consultation over hospital admission, the decision may not be appropriate or based on adequate information. Comparison of the people who die in hospital and those who die at home

[1] Williamson, J., *et. al.*, 'Old people at home: their unreported needs'.

suggests that often home conditions and circumstances are more important than nursing needs in determining admission. Yet it is doubtful whether hospital staff are adequately equipped with the social skills and the information needed to make these decisions. It seems likely, too, that other facilities—for example, homes providing basic nursing and personal care—may often be more appropriate but unavailable so that hospital is the only alternative when conditions at the person's home reach crisis level.

Hospital – general practitioner The knowledge and experience on which the decision to discharge terminally ill patients is made is even more questionable. Three-fifths of the general practitioners were critical about consultations over discharge. Lack of consultation or assessment of home circumstances and delays in communication were common complaints.

Hospital – community services There was little or no evidence of active collaboration between hospitals and other community services, and the occasions on which hospital staff had arranged community services for patients were few and far between.[1]

General practitioner – community services The mobilisation of the main community services depended largely on the general practitioner. To do this effectively he needs to be aware of patients' needs and of the services. But, as we have seen, he is not consulted about a sizeable proportion of distressing symptoms, and quite often general practitioners were apparently unaware of existing services. The importance doctors attach to community services can be judged by the fact that between 43% and 56% of them were quite prepared to accept the non-existence of bathing services and services for the care of incontinent patients.

District nurses – general practitioners About a quarter of the nurses felt that doctors did not ask for nursing help at the right time, a fifth that they did not have enough contact with the general practitioners, and rather more than half that the

[1] Hospital staff were said to have arranged for a district nurse for 5% and a home help for 3% of the people receiving these types of help.

information they were given about patients was somewhat inadequate. Attachment of nurses to general practice seemed to improve the relationship from both the doctor's and the nurse's point of view. It also meant that more of the people who died had been helped by a nurse.

Health visitors – general practitioners The potential role of health visitors in the care of dying patients did not seem to be appreciated by many general practitioners. Yet the part played by a few in the supervision and mobilisation of services could be complementary to that of the general practitioner. Obviously the effectiveness of health visitors will be severely limited if doctors do not recognise the help they can give and do not refer patients to them.

Housing The provision of suitable housing for old and ill people does not seem to be effectively linked with other social or welfare services. Local authorities give grants for improving housing amenities in certain circumstances, but they do not appear to go to old people living on their own, a third of whom have outside lavatories and no bathroom with running hot and cold water. Sheltered housing in which people receive some sort of supervision and personal care was conspicuous by its absence.[1] As more health centres are built, surely there could be scope for experimental housing projects related to such centres. The general practitioners and other community workers there should be aware of the people who need such services and should be able to provide much of the supervision and care needed. Many doctors wanted beds in hospital where they could care for some of their patients in terminal illness. It might be more appropriate for them to look after rather more of their patients in housing schemes associated with their health centre.

General practitioner – relatives Almost two-thirds of the relatives had found the patient's doctor easy to talk to and felt he had time to discuss things. Others had not found it so easy to form a satisfactory personal relationship with him. A third of the

[1] Only about 1% of the people aged 65 or more lived in housing where a warden gave some sort of supervision.

relatives had not been able to find out all they wanted to know about the deceased's illness in the detail they wanted. A quarter of the doctors were critical of relatives, feeling that they did not accept reasonable responsibility for looking after people at home. These doctors tended to be older, to have visited patients less frequently, and more often reported difficulty in obtaining hospital admissions for their patients. Their criticisms contrast rather strangely with the volume and intensity of care given by relatives and friends to many of the people who died.

Relatives – patients Three-quarters of the people who died needed some help at home during the last year of their lives. Most of the help with self care, much of the nursing care, and the bulk of the night and social care and the housework devolved on relatives and friends. Wives, husbands and daughters generally bore the brunt of this responsibility. Their descriptions of how this had affected their lives suggest that many had accepted heavy loads and responsibilities, often over quite long periods. The number of different people who helped increased with the extent of the dying person's restrictions and needs but did not increase with the length of time the person needed help. Once relatives started to look after someone they did not seem to be relieved or to get help from other relatives or friends when the need for care persisted for a long time.

When people had no husband or wife to care for them the district nurse was more likely to help them. When people who lived alone became restricted most appeared to go and live with relatives or to be admitted to hospital.

Doctor – patient – relative When someone is dying the knowledge of this may be given by a doctor to the patient, a close relative or to both; it may be withheld altogether, patients or relatives may be deliberately misled or they may realise the truth without being told. Just over a third of the people who died were thought by the people we interviewed to have known that they were dying. About three-quarters of the relatives said they had known. These proportions were similar for those who died at home and those who died in hospital. Most of the dying who were thought to have been aware of their approaching death were said not to have been told by anyone—it had been discussed directly with only 6%. Few doctors apparently felt it appropriate to tell the majority of patients this. Most relatives felt that the knowledge about the outcome was reasonably given to or withheld from the person who died, but two-fifths of the relatives who did not know themselves said they would rather have known. We can only speculate how the deceased people would react if we could ask them a similar question. Some of them, too, may have contributed to the conspiracy of silence, feeling this made it easier for their relatives and the doctors. Inevitably such constraints affect relationships. Withholding such vital information implies a willingness to assume responsibilities for a person.

And if knowledge of impending death is withheld from relatives it will mean that all their grieving has to be done after the person dies. They will not have been able to do any preparatory grieving, so their distress may be longer and more intense. The circumstances in which information is withheld from the dying and from close relations and the ethical basis for such decisions should be widely discussed, particularly in the medical curriculum. Other changes in medical education and orientation are also suggested by this study.

Redistribution of care

Although our social class analyses suggest that there is much truth in the view of death as the great equaliser, a number of suggestions emerged about ways in which care and services might be more appropriately distributed.

First, there might with advantage be a different distribution of 'cases', particularly between teaching and other hospitals. Relatively few people, 2%, die in teaching hospitals. This suggests not only that doctors are rarely confronted with death during their training but also that they do not see much of the illnesses which most often cause death. The proportion of people dying in N.H.S. hospitals was appreciably higher, three-quarters, for those dying from relatively uncommon causes such as diseases of the digestive or genito-urinary systems than it was for those dying of cancer, circulatory or respiratory diseases, between 47% and 59%. It was 38% for those with ischaemic heart disease.

Secondly, there needs to be more emphasis in medical education on caring and relieving rather than curing. The concentration in teaching hospitals, where doctors get almost all their training, on acute, short-term illness resulting in discharge inevitably orientates doctors to curing patients. The skills inculcated and admired are diagnosis and specific therapy. Yet the common medical needs today are for the relief of chronic, and common, conditions. General practitioners based in the community must be aware of this, yet there is evidence in the comments of both district nurses and relatives that some doctors are apt to lose interest when they realise that a patient is unlikely to recover. Their basic training is no doubt partly to blame, but the general impotence of the medical profession to help effectively with some problems is likely to contribute to their rejection of some patients.

So thirdly, there should be more investment in research on common symptoms and conditions, and more resources devoted to their care. Our health and social services may have partially mitigated the crude workings of the inverse care law: 'the availability of good . . . care tends to vary inversely with the need of the population served'.[1] But the law could be reformulated: the availability of good care tends to vary inversely with the number of people suffering from a condition. And we all die.

[1] Hart, Julian Tudor, 'The inverse care law'.

APPENDIX I

THE SAMPLES OF AREAS AND DEATHS

The areas

The sample areas for this study were registration districts. To select twelve areas all the registration districts in England and Wales were first divided into two groups: county and London boroughs in the first, other registration districts (combinations of municipal boroughs, urban and rural districts) in the second. Both groups were listed by region[1] and their populations summed cumulatively. The total population was divided by twelve to give a sampling fraction and a number under this was taken from a book of random numbers to give a starting point. The district which contained this number was taken as our first study area. The second and other areas were obtained by successive additions of the sampling fraction to the starting point. This gave a stratified sample of areas selected with a probability proportional to population. The areas are shown in Table A1.[2]

The deaths

The interviewing was done during the six months July–December 1969, two areas being covered in each calendar month. In order to cover deaths occurring at all times of the year, half the sample was selected from deaths which were registered three months previously and the other half from deaths registered nine months previously. Forty deaths were taken in each of the two periods in each of the twelve areas—a total of 960 in all. The plan is shown in Table A2.

The deaths were selected by the General Register Office. They took a random sample of deaths registered during the relevant period of persons aged 15 and over whose usual place of residence was in the study area.

[1] The ten regions are Northern, East and West Ridings, North Midland, Eastern, London and South-Eastern, Southern, South-Western, Wales, Midland and North-Western.

[2] By chance, no areas from three regions—East and West Ridings, North Midland and South-Western—are included in the sample.

Appendix I

TABLE A1 *Study areas*

Area	*County*	*Region*	*Population mid-1967*[a]
Teesside South[b]	Yorkshire, North Riding	Northern	272,340
Middlesbrough C.B.			154,580
Eston U.D.			40,120
Guisborough U.D. (part)			1,340
Redcar M.B.			35,960
Saltburn & Marske-by-the-Sea U.D. (Part)			10
Thornaby-on-Tees M.B.			23,450
Stokesley R.D. (part)			16,880
Barking L.B.	G.L.C.	London and South-Eastern	170,100
Hillingdon L.B.	G.L.C.	London and South-Eastern	234,470
Eastbourne C.B.	East Sussex	London and South-Eastern	66,800
Birmingham C.B.	Warwickshire	Midland	1,101,990
St Helens C.B.	Lancashire	North-Western	103,320
Northumberland North Second	Northumberland	Northern	30,040
Amble U.D.			4,980
Alnwick U.D.			7,500
Alnwick R.D.			12,320
Rothbury R.D.			5,240
Brentwood	Essex	Eastern	171,600
Brentwood U.D.			57,000
Basildon U.D.			114,600
Thanet	Kent	London and South-Eastern	136,650
Margate M.B.			49,060
Ramsgate M.B.			38,810
Sandwich M.B.			4,590
Broadstairs & St Peter's U.D.			20,300
Eastry R.D. (part)			23,890[c]

Appendix I

Area	*County*	*Region*	*Population mid-1967*[a]
Isle of Wight	Isle of Wight	Southern	98,040
Newport M.B.			19,690
Ryde M.B.			21,200
Sandown-Shanklin U.D.			13,930
Cowes U.D.			17,820
Ventnor U.D.			6,260
Isle of Wight R.D.			19,140
Bridgend	Glamorgan	Wales	171,290
Cowbridge M.B.			1,150
Maesteg U.D.			21,350
Ogmore & Garw U.D.			20,490
Bridgend U.D.			15,110
Porthcawl U.D.			12,810
Penybont R.D.			47,560
Cowbridge R.D.			21,900
Llantrisant & Llantwit Fardre R.D. (part)			30,920[c]
North-East Cheshire	Cheshire	North-Western	144,470
Bredbury & Romiley U.D.			27,620
Hazel Grove & Bramhall U.D.			34,800
Marple U.D.			23,300
Cheadle & Gatley U.D.			54,920
Disley R.D.			3,830

[a] The sample was drawn on mid-1967 figures. Mid-1968 figures have since been published and show a general increase of up to 3%. In Birmingham there was a decrease of 2½%.

[b] Middlesbrough C.B., Eston U.D., Redcar M.B. and Thornaby-on-Tees M.B. now form part of the new Teesside C.B.

[c] These populations relate to the whole of the administrative districts, although some parts fall in other registration areas.

TABLE A2 *Sampling plan*

Month of interview	*Study areas*	*Months of death registration*
July 1969	Barking L.B. Teesside South	October 1968 and April 1969
August 1969	Hillingdon L.B. North-East Cheshire	November 1968 and May 1969
September 1969	Brentwood and Basildon Bridgend	December 1968 and June 1969
October 1969	Northumberland North Second[a] Eastbourne C.B.	January 1969 and July 1969
November 1969	Birmingham C.B. Thanet	February 1969 and August 1969
December 1969	St Helens C.B. Isle of Wight	March 1969 and September 1969

[a] Northumberland North Second has such a small population that deaths registered in December 1968 and January 1969, and June and July 1969, had to be taken to give enough numbers.

Comparisons of this sample of 960 deaths with all the adult deaths in 1969 show roughly similar proportions of males (51% in the population, 53% in the sample) but the sample contains a relatively low proportion of people aged 75 or more and a high proportion of cancer deaths.

Table A3 shows the age distribution of deaths in the sample and compares it with the expected distribution calculated from all deaths in 1969. Table A4 makes the same comparison by broad cause of death. Obviously the two biases are related since deaths of people aged 75 and over are less often attributed to cancer than deaths of younger people. In 1969 the proportion of cancer deaths was 13% among those aged 75 or more, 27% among those aged 15–74.

Three possible explanations for the bias are examined—the seasonal bias in our sample of deaths, the selection of areas and the place of death.

The seasonal distribution of deaths

The bias built into the sample by taking equal numbers of deaths in all calendar months would lead to some slight under-representation of deaths of people aged 75 or more, since deaths of older people

TABLE A3 *Deaths at different ages*

	Sample of deaths		*Expected deaths*[a]	
	%	*Number*	*Number*	%
15–24	1	7	8	1
25–34	0	5	8	1
35–44	3	33	21	2
45–54	7	68	61	6
55–64	18	169	158	17
65–69	16	155	129	13
70–74	15	141	144	15
75–79	15	140	152	16
80–84	12 } 40	119 } 381	137 } 430	14 } 45
85+	13	122	141	15
Total	100	959[b]	959	100

[a] Estimated from all deaths in 1969.
[b] The age at death was illegible on one death certificate.

TABLE A4 *Cause of death*

	I.C.D. number[a]	*Sample of deaths*		*Expected deaths*[b]	
		%	*Number*	*Number*	%
Infective and parasitic	000–136	1	5	5	1
Neoplasms	140–239	27	258	197	21
Endocrine, nutritional and metabolic	240–279	1	10	11	1
Nervous system and sense organs	320–389	1	12	10	1
Circulatory	390–458	51	493	503	52
Respiratory	460–519	12	117	142	15
Digestive	520–577	2	15	23	2
Genito-urinary	580–629	2	17	14	1
Symptoms and ill-defined conditions	780–796	—	4	7	1
Accidents	E800–E999	3	27	36	4
Others	Rest	—	2	12	1
Total		100	960	960	100

[a] International Classification of Diseases—1967.
[b] Estimated from all deaths of people aged 15 and over in 1969.

form a slightly higher proportion of deaths in the 'winter' months[1] when the total number of deaths is greater. In the period October 1968–September 1969, 56% of the adult deaths occurred in six 'winter' months, 44% in the other 'summer' ones. The proportion of the adult deaths that were of people aged 75 or more were 46% in the 'winter', 44% in the 'summer'. But the estimated effect of this bias on the expected age distribution of deaths is negligible and cannot explain the much larger difference in our sample.[2]

The bias and the selection of areas

The most probable explanation for this bias lies in the selection of areas. Age distributions and mortality rates differ widely between areas. The small number of areas in the sample—twelve out of a total of 520—means that by chance the age distribution of the sample may differ appreciably from that of the total population. Data about all deaths in 1969 in the twelve study areas show that on average 42·9% of the deaths were of people aged 75 and over. This proportion is almost midway between the 40% in our sample and the 45% in England and Wales. And the sampling error calculated from our data is 2·8%,[3] which means that from our sample we would estimate the true proportion to lie between 34% and 45%.

Comparison of the observed and expected deaths of people aged 75 and over in the different areas (Table A5) shows that altogether the differences are unlikely to occur by chance: $p < 0·05$. Two areas, Barking and Hillingdon, contribute the bulk of the discrepancies.

Differences between the number of observed and expected cancer deaths in the areas are most unlikely to have occurred by chance: $p < 0·001$.

Obviously something went wrong in the selection of the sample in Hillingdon. If this area is excluded, the total chi-square for the other eleven areas is 15·37, $0·10 < p < 0·50$, but the differences in Barking and Birmingham on their own are large enough to cause some anxiety.

When these points were taken up with the Office of Population Censuses and Surveys it was found that one sub-district in Hillingdon which consisted solely of hospital premises had been excluded from the sample. This suggested that we should examine the distribution

[1] November–April inclusive.

[2] Theoretically we would expect 433 of the 960 deaths to be of people aged 75 and over if deaths had been sampled in proportion to the number occurring in winter and summer, compared with 432 by taking equal numbers in winter and summer.

[3] See Appendix VIII.

TABLE A5 *Variations between areas*

	Deaths of people aged 75 and over			Cancer deaths		
	Observed	Expected[a]	χ^2	Observed	Expected[a]	χ^2
Teesside South[b]	30	29·9	—	17	16·2	0·05
Barking	17	30·8	10·05	30	20·9	5·36
Hillingdon	21	33·0	7·42	36	18·3	22·20
Eastbourne	39	44·7	1·65	18	17·3	0·04
Birmingham	26	32·3	2·06	26	17·3	5·58
St Helens	25	29·6	1·13	15	15·2	—
Brentwood	42	39·2	0·39	22	17·4	1·55
Thanet	38	40·5	0·31	21	17·7	0·79
Isle of Wight	38	40·2	0·24	20	15·8	1·39
Bridgend	32	30·5	0·12	13	14·7	0·24
North-East Cheshire	32	35·2	0·54	21	19·6	0·13
Northumberland North Second	41	38·7	0·27	19	17·2	0·24
Total	381	424·6	24·18	258	207·6	37·57

[a] Calculated on data for 1969 supplied by the Office of Population Censuses and Surveys.
[b] Figures for Teesside C.B. used for comparisons.

of the sample by place of death, which we had not done earlier because no figures are published on the place of death by age. However, the Office of Population Censuses and Surveys had made an analysis of the place of death by age and cause in 1965. This is considered next.

Place of death

The proportion of deaths occurring in different places did not change greatly between 1965 and 1969, and in 1965 the place of death for adults aged 15 and over was similar to that for all deaths, so it seems reasonable to compare the place of death in our sample with the figures for all deaths in 1969. This is done in Table A6. The sample included a low proportion of hospital deaths and a correspondingly high proportion of home deaths. If Hillingdon is excluded the distribution is not materially altered; if anything, the discrepancy is greater. (Fifty-one per cent of the sample of deaths from Hillingdon occurred in N.H.S. non-psychiatric hospitals.)

TABLE A6 *Place of death*

	1965				
	Adults 15 & over	*All deaths*	*1969 all deaths*	*Sample all areas*	*Sample excluding Hillingdon*
	%	%	%	%	%
Mental hospital or psychiatric institution	3	3	3	3	3
Other N.H.S. hospital or institution for care of sick	47	48	51	44	43
Private nursing home or hospital	2	2	3	4	4
Other institutions	4	4	3	3	3
Own home	39	38	35	40	40
Elsewhere	5	5	5	6	7
Number of deaths (=100%)	527,763	549,379	579,378	960	880

This bias in the place of death seems unrelated to the bias with age and cause of death. Figures for 1965 show that people aged 15–74 were rather more likely to die in hospital but rather less likely to die in private nursing homes or other institutions than those aged 75 or over. Adults who died of cancer were slightly more likely than adults dying of other conditions to die in hospital (Table A7).

It would seem, therefore, that this is an additional bias. Again, it probably results from the small number of areas chosen, as there were wide variations in the place of death between areas. The estimated range for the proportion of home deaths calculated from our sampling error is from 35% to 45%.

The effects of the biases

The main effects of the age and cause of death bias is that the sample contains an *excess* of young (under 75) cancer deaths—21% compared with 15% in England and Wales in 1969—and a deficit of deaths from other causes of people aged 75 or more, 34% against 39%. (There was no difference between the sample as drawn and the deaths for whom a main interview was completed on this.)

TABLE A7 *Place of death by age and cause of death in 1965*

	Deaths aged 15–74	Deaths aged 75 or more	Adults dying of	
			Cancer	Other causes
Place of death	%	%	%	%
Mental hospital or psychiatric institution	3	4	1	4
Other N.H.S. hospital or institution for care of the sick	50	43	54	45
Private nursing home or hospital	1	4	4	2
Other institutions	1	7	1	4
Own home	38	39	37	39
Elsewhere	7	3	3	6
Number of deaths (=100%)	291,508	236,255	106,844	420,919

Reweighting to correct for this bias shows that the sample has an excess of married and a deficit of widowed people (Table A8).[1] (The reweighted proportions are similar to the distribution among all adult deaths.) As a result of this, rather more interviews were done with widows and widowers than would be expected, 39% against 36%. Similar analyses by sex, social class, restrictions, symptoms, help needed and help given by professionals and by relatives and friends showed that this bias did not have a significant effect on any of these.

In the main report no attempt has therefore been made to correct for the biases.

The response

Because data from the death certificate were available for all the deaths in our sample it is possible to see whether the response rate varied with the information recorded on the death certificate. Table A9 shows the variation in response rate by the age, sex and social class of occupation of the deceased.

[1] This was done by cross-analysing marital status for those under and over 75 and those dying of cancer and other causes and then reweighting by the correct instead of observed proportions in these groups.

TABLE A8 *Effect of bias on marital status*

	Sample interviewed	*Reweighted to correct for bias*	*Among adult deaths in England and Wales*
Marital status	%	%	%
Single	12	12	12
Married	52	49	49
Widowed, divorced or separated	36	39	39
Number of deaths (=100%)	772		555,788

There was no significant variation in the response rate with the sex or age of the deceased. With social class the response rate was poor when the data about occupation were inadequate. In spite of the apparently good response in the professional class (which is based on small numbers and is not a statistically significant difference) the response rate was better among the working class than the middle class. Table A10 shows that the response varied by area and was better in the north than in the south.[1] Another study reported similar north/south differences.[2]

Cross-analyses of social class and north/south areas shows that the response rate was lowest, 74%, among the middle class in the south. It was 84% among the working class in the south and did not differ between the middle and working class in the north.

There was no significant variation in the response rate with the cause of death. Table A11 shows that a successful interview was more often obtained when a husband, wife, son or daughter registered the death than when it was another person or relative. This suggests that we may have been more likely to get a completed interview when there was a close relative living near or taking an interest in the deceased.

Analysis by place of death in Table A12 suggests that the response rate may have been rather higher when the person died in his own or someone else's home than when he died in a hospital, institution or elsewhere. This difference, combined with that in the person registering the death, suggests that isolated persons with no close relatives to look after them may be under-represented in the sample.

[1] The Bristol–Wash line was taken as the dividing line.

[2] See Cartwright, Ann, *Human Relations and Hospital Care*, p. 213.

TABLE A9 *Variation in response with sex, age and social class of occupation of the person who died*

	Proportion for which main questionnaire completed		Number of deaths (=100%)
Sex			
Male	83%		505
Female	80%		455
Age[a]			
15–24	78% (15–44 combined)		45
25–34			
35–44			
45–54	81%		68
55–64	87%		168
65–69	83%		155
70–74	78%		142
75–79	79%		140
80–84	84%		119
85+	80%		122
Social class of occupation[b]			
I Professional	90%	78% (I–III Non-manual)	30
II Intermediate	77%		152
III Skilled Non-manual	76%		115
Manual	84%	85% (III Manual–V)	309
IV Semi-skilled	87%		204
V Unskilled	86%		98
Not classified	65%		52
Total sample	82%		960

[a] One, for whom the date was illegible on the death certificate, was not classified by age.

[b] Eleven people who were in the forces or students could not be classified by social class of occupation. For the other 41 not classified the information was inadequate.

Is there any evidence about this from the deaths for which we collected only partial information?

The partial responders

The small number, thirty-two, of people for whom partial, but not complete, information was collected can be used to improve our

TABLE A10 *Variation in response with area*

	Proportion for which main questionnaire completed		*Number of deaths (=100%)*
Northumberland	88%	84%	80
Teesside South	88%		80
St Helens	83%		80
North-East Cheshire	81%		80
Birmingham	85%		80
Bridgend	81%		80
Brentwood and Basildon	84%	79%	80
Hillingdon	73%		80
Barking	90%		80
Thanet	74%		80
Eastbourne	79%		80
Isle of Wight	78%		80
Total sample	82%		960

TABLE A11 *Variation in response with person who registered death*

Relationship to dead person of person who registered death[a]	*Proportion for which main questionnaire completed*	*Number of deaths (=100%)*
Husband or wife	86%	215
Son or daughter	83%	378
Other relative	78%	241
Other person[b]	79%	90
Coroner	76%	33
Total sample	82%	957[a]

[a] Inadequate information was recorded on three death certificates.
Neighbours, friends, officials of institution or undertakers.

TABLE A I 2 *Variation in response with place of death*

Place of death	*Proportion for which main questionnaire completed*	*Number of deaths (=100%)*
Mental hospital or psychiatric institution	81%	31
Other N.H.S. hospital or institution for the care of the sick	80%	420
Private nursing home	78%	40
Other institution	83%	29
Own home	85%	381
Other address	90%	30
Elsewhere[a]	76%	29

[a] In street, ambulance, etc.

TABLE A I 3 *Comparison of successes, failures and partial successes*

	Successes	*Partial successes*	*Failures*	*Total*
Proportion of women	47%	66%	47%	47%
Proportion aged 75 or more	40%	38%	41%	40%
Proportion dying in own home	41%	25%	36%	40%
Proportion dying of cancer	27%	22%	25%	27%
Death registered by:	%	%	%	%
Spouse	24	3	21	23
Son/daughter	40	28	38	40
Other relative	24	35	29	25
Other person	9	25	8	9
Coroner	3	9	4	3
Proportion middle class[a]	31%	32%	43%	33%
Proportion for whom the person who registered the death lived in the same household as the dead person[b]	46%	28%	47%	45%
Number of deaths (=100%)[c]	785	32	143	960

[a] Excluding people in the forces.

[b] Excluding deaths registered by the coroner.

[c] Those for whom inadequate information was obtained have been excluded when calculating percentages.

estimates in some respects. But data from the death certificates suggest that, in a number of ways, the people for whom we got no information were more like those for whom we got complete

TABLE A14 *Effect of including the partial successes*

	Partial successes	*Complete successes*	*Total-any successes*
Marital status of person who died	%	%	%
Married	26	52	51
Single	35	12	13
Widowed	39	34	34
Divorced or separated	—	2	2
Household composition	%	%	%
On own	25	15	15
With spouse or others of same or older generation only	29	37	37
With relatives of younger generation	25	42	41
With unrelated people or in guesthouse	21	6	7
Death	%	%	%
Expected	44	56	55
Unexpected	44	10	12
Neither expected nor unexpected	12	34	33
How long in hospital or institution before died there	%	%	%
Did not die in hospital or institution	39	49	48
Less than a month	37	29	30
A month but less than a year	10	13	13
A year or more	14	9	9
Restricted	%	%	%
Bedridden or confined mainly to bed for 3 months or more	15	21	21
Other restriction for 3 months or more	42	46	46
Restricted for less than 3 months	15	16	16
Not restricted	28	17	17
Number of deaths (=100%)[a]	32	785	817

Those for whom inadequate information was obtained have been excluded when the percentages were calculated.

interviews than those for whom we collected only partial data. This is illustrated in Table A13.

There was no difference between the three groups in the proportion aged 75 or more or in the proportion dying of cancer. The partial successes were more like the failures in relation to dying at home and more like the successes in relation to class. But the deaths of the partial successes were more likely to have been registered by someone who was not a relative and by someone who did not live at the same address than either the successes or failures. These comparisons suggest it would be unwise to assume that the failures were more like the partial successes than the successes.

Comparing information collected for the partial successes (in Table A14) it appears that the person who died was more often single and rather more often lived with unrelated people. This is further evidence that the socially isolated may be under-represented in our completed interviews. However, inclusion of the partial responders did not make any significant difference to our sample estimates. They have not been included in the main report.

APPENDIX II

THE SAMPLE OF GENERAL PRACTITIONERS

There are three problems, or sources of bias, about the sample of general practitioners. The first is related to the way the areas were chosen, the second to the way doctors were chosen within the areas, and the third to their response rate.

Areas

The areas were selected with probability proportional to population. Once this has been done equal weight should be attached to each of the areas to give a random sample.[1] We did this for our sample of deaths by taking equal numbers in the twelve areas, but because we obtained our sample of general practitioners through the deaths and because the areas varied so much in population size (from 30,040 to 1,101,990), the number of different doctors reported in the areas varied from fifteen in Northumberland to fifty-five in Birmingham. The result is that doctors from the larger areas are over-represented.

One way to correct this bias is by weighting each doctor by the number of deaths of his patients in our sample, so that doctors with one death in the sample are included once, with two twice, etc. The distribution is given in Table A15. It shows, for example, that four doctors were each reported for six deaths. These four doctors just appear once in the unweighted sample, but are each given a weight of six in the weighted sample, making a total of twenty-four because twenty-four patients who died had these doctors.

Table A16 shows the effect of this reweighting on a number of characteristics for which information was available from the Department of Health and Social Security.[2] The first column shows the distribution among the reported doctors (each doctor being included once, irrespective of the number of deaths of his patients in the sample), and the second column the distribution among the patients'

[1] A random sample means, statistically, that each unit has an equal chance of being selected.

[2] Sixteen, 4%, of the 427 doctors reported could not be traced in the Department records, mainly because people gave us inadequate information.

TABLE A15 *Number of patients with the same doctor*

Number of patients with the same doctor	*Number of doctors*	*Number of patients*
1	267	267
2	97	194
3	40	120
4	8	32
5	8	40
6	4	24
7	—	—
8	—	—
9	2	18
10	1	10
Total	427	705[a]

[a] When the patient had been in a hospital or institution for a year or more we did not ask about his doctor. This happened 81 times. For another 31 the doctor could not be traced.

doctors with doctors reweighted according to the number of their patients in the sample of deaths. None of the differences are significant.

Table A17 shows some of the answers on the survey for the doctors who participated, comparing the unweighted sample with the weighted one. Again there were no significant differences. The unweighted sample of reported doctors has generally been used in the report for analyses which involve doctors only. Cross-analyses of patients' and doctors' characteristics are of course based on the weighted sample.

Selection within areas

The general practitioners in our study are the doctors of a randomly selected sample of people who died in a particular period in England and Wales.

Other implications besides the one already discussed are:

1. Doctors who work mainly or entirely with young people or children will be under-represented or missing. Those with a high proportion of elderly patients have a greater chance of being included.

TABLE A16 *Comparison of selected doctors with weighted sample of patients' doctors (data from Department of Health and Social Security)*

	Reported doctors	*Patients' doctors (weighted sample)*
Sex	%	%
Men	95	96
Women	5	4
Age	%	%
Under 35	8	8
35–44	27	26
45–54	33	37
55–64	26	25
65+	6	4
Number of principals	%	%
One	22	21
Two	25	24
Three	29	32
Four	15	15
Five or more	9	8
Eligible for rural practice payments	%	%
Yes	10	14
No	90	86
Type of area	%	%
Designated	48	42
Intermediate	13	18
Open	34	32
Restricted	5	8
Eligible for group practice payments	%	%
Yes	53	56
No	47	44
Numbers on which percentages based[a]	427	705

[a] Those for whom inadequate information was obtained have been excluded when calculating percentages.

2. Doctors with large numbers of patients will have a greater chance of being included than doctors with small numbers, since the chance of being included is related to the number of patients who died.

TABLE A17 *Comparison of selected doctors with weighted sample of patients' doctors (survey data)*

	Reported doctors	*Patients' doctors (weighted sample)*
Proportion thinking that in their area they need more:		
Short-term beds	47%	47%
Chronic hospital beds	86%	86%
Geriatric beds	89%	90%
Mental hospital places	34%	35%
District nurse services	24%	21%
Home help services	55%	53%
Proportion regarding home help service as:	%	%
Adequate	24	28
Rather inadequate	49	44
Very inadequate	27	28
Proportion who usually find it easy to get admission into a suitable N.H.S. institution for:		
A young patient with a short-term terminal illness	71%	71%
An old patient with a short-term terminal illness	28%	28%
An old patient likely to need long-term nursing care	10%	11%
A young patient likely to need long-term nursing care	29%	29%
An old patient with an acute infection	58%	58%
Approximate number of N.H.S. patients they look after:	%	%
Under 2,000	8	7
2,000–2,499	18	20
2,500–2,999	31	32
3,000–3,499	29	28
3,500+	14	13
Number of doctors (=100%)[a]	323	550

[a] Small numbers for whom inadequate information was obtained have been excluded when the percentages were calculated.

3. Doctors of patients under-represented in our sample of deaths, because of failure to obtain an interview, will be likely to be under-represented in our sample of doctors. So doctors caring for a high proportion of socially isolated people may be inadequately represented. The biases in the sample of deaths may also affect the sample of doctors.

TABLE A18 *Comparison of sample of general practitioners with national data*

	Sample of reported doctors	*England and Wales 1968*[a]
Sex	%	%
Male	95	90
Female	5	10
Age	%	%
Under 35	8	13
35–44	27	32
45–54	33	30
55–64	26	18
65+	6	7
Number of principals	%	%
One	22	23
Two	25	27
Three	29	26
Four	15	14
Five or more	9	10
Type of area	%	%
Designated	48	33
Intermediate	13	17
Open	34	40
Restricted	5	10
Number of doctors (=100%)	427[b]	19,923[c]

[a] Annual Report of the Department of Health and Social Security for the Year 1968, pp. 86–90. Figures available for 1969 do not include Wales.

[b] Those for whom inadequate information was obtained have been excluded when calculating percentages.

[c] The base varied in practice being 19,970 for the type of area. This included principals providing restricted services only.

Table A18 compares the doctors in our sample with the general practitioner principals in England and Wales. The sample contains relatively few women doctors and a comparatively high proportion of older doctors aged 55 or more. This is probably because women doctors tend to be more involved with the care of children and with maternity work and older doctors tend to have older patients.[1] From the point of view of this study these 'biases' are reasonable, in the sense that they suggest our sample is weighted towards doctors caring for patients who are likely to die. There was little difference in the size of partnerships, but the sample contains a high proportion of doctors working in designated areas. This bias is probably the result of the small number of areas. The majority of doctors in five of our study areas—Barking, Teesside, Brentwood and Basildon, Birmingham and St Helens—worked in designated areas.

The response

We asked the name of the general practitioner for the 737 people who had died but had not been in a hospital or institution for all the twelve months before they died. Two respondents refused to tell us the name and another twenty-nine gave us inadequate or incorrect information so that we were unable to trace the doctors. Sixteen, 4%, of the doctors they told us about had died, retired or were no longer working in the areas. Of the remaining 411 doctors 323, 79%, were interviewed or filled in a postal questionnaire. Table A19 shows the doctors' response from the point of view of both doctors and patients who died.

We tried to interview a random fifth of the doctors and sent postal questionnaires to the other four-fifths. The response rate was 84% in the first group, 77% in the second. Such a difference might arise by chance, and included in the 84% response rate of those we tried to interview are 6% who were not prepared to be interviewed but who completed postal questionnaires.

Analysis of the response rate with the various characteristics such as age, sex, number of principals in partnership and type of area available for all doctors from the Department of Health and Social Security revealed no significant differences.

We can also see whether the people we interviewed varied in their views of the general practitioners who responded and those who did not, and whether there was any difference in the care the doctors were said to have given the people who died.

[1] See Cartwright, Ann, *Patients and their Doctors*, pp. 168 and 183.

TABLE A19 *Response of general practitioners*

	Patients	*Doctors*
Doctor:		
Interviewed	550 (Interviewed and Completed postal questionnaire combined)	67
Completed postal questionnaire		256 (total 323)
Refused or did not reply[a]	136	88
Retired, moved or died	19	16
Untraced or respondent refused to give name of doctor	31	—
Not asked about because long-term institutional death	81	—
Total	817	427

[a] After three reminders.

There was no difference between the groups in their place of death, and the differences shown in Table A20 in the numbers of consultations and home visits might have occurred by chance. But, if anything, the doctors who refused or did not reply had less contact with the patients who died than those who co-operated, and their patients were less likely to have been visited by a district nurse. Respondents more often felt the doctor did not have time to discuss things when he failed to reply to the questionnaire, but they were no less likely to feel he was easy to talk to. A higher proportion said they knew what was wrong with the deceased when the doctor co-operated (51%) than when he did not (38%) and more of them said they got most of their information from the deceased's general practitioner: 48% against 37%.

These findings suggest that the general practitioners who responded may have a somewhat closer relationship with their patients and their patients' families than those who did not. They seem to be more willing to spend time both filling in questionnaires and talking to patients' relatives.

Summary

Although there are three sources of bias affecting the sample of general practitioners in this study, comparisons suggest that the most important is our failure to obtain information about 21% of the doctors approached. Information from patients' relatives suggests that the failure rate may have been higher among doctors with a less good relationship with patients.

TABLE A20 *Some comparisons of data about general practitioner care when doctors collaborated on the study and when they did not*

	Doctor collaborated	*Doctor refused or did not reply*	*Other failure*
Number of home visits in year before death[a]	%	%	%
0	7	11	10
1–10	49	55	54
10+	44	34	36
Relatives felt doctor had time to discuss things	%	%	%
Yes	71	64	60
No	14	24	25
Uncertain	15	12	15
Relatives felt doctor easy to talk to	%	%	%
Yes	76	73	(79)
No	13	16	(21)
Uncertain	11	11	(—)
Person who died visited by district nurse[b]	%	%	%
Yes	39	29	22
No	61	71	78
Consultations in year before death	%	%	%
0	3	5	16
1–4	21	27	13
5–9	20	22	16
10+	56	46	55
Number of deaths[c]	533	132	48

[a] Excluding those with no consultation.
[b] Those who died unexpectedly under the age of 65 have been excluded.
[c] Excluding those in hospital or institution for a year or more before they died. Those for whom inadequate information was available or to whom the question did not apply have been excluded when calculating percentages.
Percentages in brackets are based on less than 20 people.

APPENDIX III

THE SAMPLE OF DISTRICT NURSES AND HEALTH VISITORS

The Medical Officers of Health covering all twelve of our study areas agreed that we could approach the district nurses and health visitors working there. Five hundred and thirty-two district nurses were identified and 508, 95%, interviewed. There were also seventy-six health visitors involved in the care of dying or bereaved people and seventy-five of these were interviewed. The problem of non-response is therefore small. In addition, there was no problem of selecting a sample within the study areas—all those working there were included; the only difficulty was in the study areas which were part of a local health authority area. For these we needed to identify the district nurses and health visitors covering the study areas.

As areas were chosen with a probability proportional to population, there is the problem that nurses in larger areas had a greater chance of being in the sample than nurses in smaller areas, and the fact that all the nurses in an area were included increases the effect of this bias. In the area with the smallest population, Northumberland North Second (population 30,040) we interviewed twelve district nurses; in the largest, Birmingham (population 1,101,990), 209.

There were wide variations between the areas in the proportion of district nurses attached to general practitioners and in the views of the nurses on various services and their relationship with them. A number of these are shown in Table A21, which lists the study areas in order of their population. No clear trends emerged, so no attempt has been made to correct for this bias.

TABLE A21 *Variation in district nurses' work and views in study areas*

Area (Listed by size of population)	*Proportion attached to a general practice*	*Proportion feeling contact with hospital generally adequate*	*Proportion describing home help service in area as adequate*	*Proportion finding general practitioners ask for their help at about right time*	*Proportion feeling they are able to give enough time to terminally ill*	*Number of district nurses*[a] (=100%)
Small						
Northumberland (N. Second)	(50%)	(58%)	(42%)	(75%)	(83%)	12
Eastbourne	60%	25%	8%	63%	36%	25
Isle of Wight	19%	46%	15%	54%	56%	27
St Helens	(6%)	(44%)	(41%)	(88%)	(47%)	17
Thanet	57%	22%	57%	70%	61%	23
NE. Cheshire	26%	44%	18%	65%	26%	23
Barking	0%	31%	33%	54%	22%	27
Bridgend	76%	14%	34%	4%	52%	29
Brentwood	13%	26%	4%	57%	46%	23
Hillingdon	11%	34%	22%	47%	26%	36
Teesside	65%	47%	29%	76%	27%	57
Birmingham	81%	26%	11%	78%	30%	209
Large						
All district nurses in sample	56%	32%	20%	66%	36%	508

[a] Small numbers for whom inadequate information was obtained have been omitted when the percentages were calculated. Percentages in brackets are based on less than 20 people.

APPENDIX IV

COMPARISON OF DATA FROM INTERVIEWS AND DEATH CERTIFICATES

Three items of information recorded on the death certificate were asked about at the interview and coded independently—cause of death, age at time of death and place of death. Data about occupation were also recorded on the death certificate, and from these social class was coded and compared with information collected at the interview for some of the people who died.

Cause of death

The underlying cause of death had already been coded by the G.R.O. on the death certificate. If we compare the broad classification[1] with the cause of death reported by the relative (or other respondent) and coded in the same way, we find that the distributions are roughly similar except that relatives attributed fewer

TABLE A22 *Underlying cause of death—distributions*

	Death certificate	*Relatives*
	%	%
Neoplasm	27	27
Circulatory	51	46
Respiratory	12	11
Digestive	2	2
Accident	3	3
Old age, senility	—	5
Other	5	6
Number of deaths (=100%)	785	756

[1] Into neoplasms/circulatory/ respiratory/digestive/accidents/senility and other causes.

TABLE A23 *Underlying cause – cross-analysis*

Relative's diagnosis	*Underlying cause on death certificate*							
	Neoplasm	*Circulatory*	*Respiratory*	*Digestive*	*Accident*	*Old age senility*	*Other*	*Total*
Neoplasm	192	4	3	2	—	—	1	202
Circulatory	8	304	23	1	6	—	9	351
Respiratory	5	18	56	—	—	—	5	84
Digestive	4	4	2	5	—	—	1	16
Accident	1	7	1	—	13	—	2	24
Old age, senility	1	28	1	—	—	2	4	36
Other	2	16	6	4	1	—	14	43
Not known	2	18	5	—	1	—	3	29
Total	215	399	97	12	21	2	39	785

deaths to circulatory disease and more to old age or senility, which was recorded as a cause of death on less than 1% of the death certificates. This is shown in Table A22. Relatives could not give a 'diagnosis' for 4% of the deaths.

The two diagnoses fell into the same broad category in 78% of cases. Table A23 gives the numbers in the cross-analysis.

Agreement was best over *neoplasms*. When the relatives gave this as the cause of death it agreed with the diagnosis on the death certificate in 95% of instances. When the respondent said the person died of cancer but this was not coded as the main cause of death on the death certificate it was mentioned there as an additional cause in six out of the ten instances. Conversely in the twenty-three cases recorded as cancer on the death certificate but not given as the main cause at the interview ten respondents mentioned this as a contributory cause.

Two main sources of discrepancies in the broad classification were accidents and '*senility or old age*'. The majority of deaths described by the relatives as being due to senility or old age were attributed by the doctors to diseases of the circulatory system (78%).

Accidents were regarded by relatives as the cause of death for twenty-four people and by doctors for twenty-one but they agreed for only thirteen. Both doctors and relatives attributed most of the other 'accidents' to circulatory conditions.

The other main disagreement was the division between *circulatory* and *respiratory* conditions. One quarter of the deaths diagnosed by doctors as respiratory were regarded by the relatives as circulatory, and a fifth of the deaths regarded by relatives as respiratory were diagnosed by doctors as circulatory.

Usually, the cause of death from the death certificate is used in the report.

Age at death

The age at death is recorded on the death certificate, and this was coded into the groups 15–24, 25–34, 35–44, 45–54, 55–64, 65–9, 70–4, 75–9, 80–4, 85+. At the interview we asked the respondent first how old the deceased was when he died (this was coded by the interviewer into one of the ten groups) and then whether he could give us the exact date of the dead person's birth.

The age of death was illegible on one death certificate, and two respondents said they did not know how old the deceased was when he died. Comparison of the data from the two sources for the other 782 deaths shows:

	Number	%
Agreement on the group	732	93·6
Interview one group older	19	2·4
Interview one group younger	28	3·6
Interview two or more groups older	2	0·3
Interview two or more groups younger	1	0·1
Total	782	100·0

There was serious disagreement in 0·4% of the deaths and no evidence of a bias in one direction rather than another among those not falling in the same category.

The three instances in which there was disagreement by more than one category were as shown in Table A24.

TABLE A24 *Disagreements on age*

Interview data			*Death certificate*			
Age group	*Date of birth*	*Respondent*	*Age*	*Date of death*	*Date of birth*	*Informant*
75–79	———	Nurse at hospital	90	18.6.69	16.4.79	Official at hospital
75–79	—.5.—	Sister-in-law	69	3.12.68	22.4.99	Nephew
55–64	23.9.?	Wife	44	25.6.69	18.9.24	Wife

In the first two it seems likely that the data on the death certificate were more reliable because the date of birth was recorded. In the third case the wife had registered the death and was interviewed. At the interview she said her husband had told her he would be 45 next birthday but the Social Security people had informed her that he was born in 1913—which would make him 55 or 56 at the time of his death.

In the analysis the age recorded on the *death certificate* is used.

Place of death

The place of death was recorded on the death certificate and had been classified into the groups described in Chapter 4. At the interview the respondent was asked where the deceased died and this was classified by whether it was a hospital, other institution,[1] the

[1] This was left to the respondent.

deceased's own home, another person's home or elsewhere (e.g. in the road, dead on arrival at hospital, etc.).

Table A25 shows the relationship between these two classifications.

TABLE A25 *Place of death from interview and death certificate data*

	Interview					*Total*
	Hospital	*Other institution*	*Own home*	*Other person's home*	*Elsewhere*	
Death certificate:						
Mental hospital or psychiatric institution	24	1	—	—	—	25
Other N.H.S. hospital	321	1	3	—	9	334
Private hospital or nursing home	14	17	—	—	—	31
Permanent residence of an institutional nature	5	17	2	—	—	24
Own home	—	2	313	6	1	322
Elsewhere	1	1	10	17	20	49
Total	365	39	328	23	30	785

There was complete agreement between the two classifications in 93% of the deaths. (That is taking mental institutions or psychiatric hospitals as hospitals, and private nursing homes and permanent places of residence of an institutional nature as 'other institutions'.) If all types of institution are taken together, the agreement is 96%, since at the interview private nursing homes and permanent residences of an institutional nature were often described as hospitals. The main discrepancies that remain include the nine instances in which a hospital was recorded on the death certificate but 'elsewhere' at the interview. Eight of the interview respondents thought the person died before they got to hospital, the other said he had died in the outpatient department while attending for X-ray. In the same way six people were thought to have died at home before being taken to hospital but were recorded on the death certificate as dying elsewhere because they were 'dead on arrival at the hospital'. The discrepancies for the other four out of the ten people said at the interview to have died at their own home but recorded on the death certificate as dying elsewhere arose from uncertainty about their home. Two were said by respondents to have been living with their children and their families when they died, but they had been doing so for less than a year and their previous address appeared to have been recorded on the death certificate. Another person had been living with her sister for between one and two years; her usual address on the death certificate was in the same road but at a different number from the address where she was recorded as dying. The fourth had lived with her two sisters for over fifty years but died 'at our other home in Wales' where she was on holiday.

Six people were recorded on the death certificate as dying in their own home, but at the interview the respondent said they died at another person's home, usually theirs. For four of the six the deceased person had apparently been living there 'permanently' but not for many years.

> 'We took her in when the cousin she was living with died.' (Niece, had been living there between two and five years.)

But two of the six seemed less permanently established.

> 'I was paying rent for his house. I told him to get out of it but he wouldn't—said he'd go back.' (Daughter with whom the person had been living for less than a year before his death).

The other, whose husband had died within the last year and who had spent much of the time since then in hospital, had been in her sister's home for a two weeks' holiday when she died, but the sister said she would have returned to an old peoples' home.

The three people recorded on the death certificate as dying in hospital but said at the interview to have died at home had all been certified by the coroner. In two the person had, according to the person we interviewed, been dead for over a day before they were found and taken to hospital for investigation. About the third death the widow had apparently misled us. She said her husband died of arteriosclerosis and had suffered from acute depression and insomnia. He died at home but had been in hospital earlier in the year. He came home less than a month before he died. On the death certificate it said that he died in hospital from a shotgun wound to the head. He shot himself while the balance of his mind was disturbed through ill health and depression.

Other discrepancies, apart from those in which institutions were classified differently, are described below:

Appendix IV

Death Certificate	*Interview*	*Details*
Permanent institution	Own home	Died in a community of monks where he had lived for over fifty years.
Permanent institution	Own home	Died in a convent where she had lived for over twenty years.
Elsewhere	Hospital	Dead on arrival at hospital according to the death certificate. At the interview it was reported that he had been in hospital less than twenty-four hours—'if he wasn't dead already'.
Own home	Elsewhere	At the interview it was reported that he died 'at the rent office a little way down the road of heart failure'.
Own home	Other institution	Sister-in-law said at the interview that she died in a nursing home where she had lived for between two and five years. The matron of the nursing home was not willing to be interviewed. The address of the matron was the same as that of the place of death on the death certificate.
Own home	Other institution	The interview was with a charge attendant at the welfare home where the person was said to have lived for between two and five years.
Elsewhere	Other institution	At the interview his brother said he died in a nursing home where he had been for between a week and a month.

In the last three instances the place of death on the death certificate was just an ordinary address.

For many analyses the place of death reported at interview is used, but the type of institution is taken from the death certificate data.

Appendix IV

Sex

On one death certificate the sex appeared to have been wrongly recorded. The name was James ———, the sex was recorded as 'female', and under cause of death 'barbiturate poisoning—he killed himself'. This has been included as a male death.

Social class

The last full-time occupation of the deceased person is recorded on the death certificate, the previous occupation if he had retired, and the husband's occupation if the deceased was a married or widowed woman. The occupation was classified according to the Registrar General's Classification of Occupations (1966) into six groups—the five social classes distinguished by the Registrar General, but with his social class III, skilled occupations, subdivided into non-manual and manual.

At the interview information was collected about the dead person's main job unless the person was a housewife and had not worked for ten years or more or had been in a hospital or institution for a year or more before death. Information was also collected about the respondent's current occupation if he was a man under 65, or a single woman under 60, about his main occupation if he was a man aged 65 or more, or a single woman of 60 or more, or about the husband's main occupation if the respondent was a woman who was or had been married (but not to the deceased, as in that case the information would already have been obtained). The occupations obtained at the interview were coded in the same way as those recorded on the death certificate.

Table A26 compares the social class distribution of the deceased's main occupation from the interview with that of the occupation on the death certificate. Slightly more were classified as middle-class (professional, intermediate or skilled non-manual) from the interview data than from the death certificate. But for married and widowed women we are comparing different information.

A cross-analysis was done for men and women separately. This showed complete agreement for 71% of the men and some agreement, including those just one category different, for 90%. As expected, the 'agreement' for women was much less good—47% showed complete agreement, 31% differed by one category; 22% by more than one.[1]

When the comparison is made for single women (on the basis of

[1] Students, people in the armed forces and those for whom information was not recorded have been excluded from these comparisons.

their own occupations) and married women whose husbands we interviewed (on the basis of the husband's occupation), the agreement is much closer than for all women together: complete in 75%, one out in 18%.

Taking the men's occupation, the interview data seemed to allot them to a higher social class than the death certificate data. Sixty-one

TABLE A26 *Social class—distributions*

	Interview		*Death certificate*	
Social class:	%		%	
I—Professional	3	37	4	32
II—Intermediate	21		16	
III—Skilled—non-manual	13		12	
III—Skilled—manual	31		34	
IV—Partly skilled	24		23	
V—Unskilled	8		11	
Number of deaths for which information available (=100%)	451		751	

were placed higher on the social class scale by the occupation recorded at the interview than on the death certificate, thirty the other way round.

In the report, data from the death certificate are used. Social class could be classified from the information there for 96% of the deaths. In 1% the occupation was given as student or armed forces and in 3% the description of occupation seemed inadequate.

APPENDIX V

DATA FROM DIFFERENT TYPES OF RESPONDENT

We tried to interview the person who could tell us most about the dead person's life in the last year. How successful were we? At the end of the interview, on the basis of all her knowledge of the circumstances, the interviewer was asked to assess whether the person interviewed was the most appropriate person or not. For three-quarters of the deaths our informant was felt to be the only appropriate person to interview. In a fifth the informant was judged to be one of two or more who were equally appropriate. For less than one in twenty, 4%, the interviewer felt it would have been more appropriate to have talked to someone else. The proportion in which they felt this was less than 1% when the husband or wife was interviewed, 3% when it was son or daughter, 10% when it was another relative, and 10% when it was an unrelated person.

In the main part of the report we showed that 69% of the interviews were with husbands, wives, sons or daughters. This proportion was higher, 73%, when the person who died was a man than when it was a woman, 63%. Table A27 shows how the respondent varied with the age of the person who died.

The older the person the less likely we were to be able to interview their husband or wife and the more likely to interview a son or daughter, but the latter did not entirely compensate for the former so we were less likely to see a close relative as the person became older and less likely to see someone in the same household. The way the respondent varied for people who had lived in different types of household is shown in Table A28. Friends, neighbours or officials of institutions were seen for about three-quarters of those who had lived with people other than relatives and for a fifth of those living on their own.

Variations in the respondent with the place of death are shown in Table A29. When the persons died in their own homes our respondent was a husband, wife, son or daughter for 78% of the interviews. This proportion was rather less, 67%, when they died in a hospital and much less, 30%, when they died in an institution.

TABLE A27 *Respondent and age of person who died*

	Age at time of death								*All ages*
	15–44	45–54	55–64	65–69	70–74	75–79	80–84	85+	
	%	%	%	%	%	%	%	%	%
Husband or wife	69 } 75	73 } 82	57 } 77	51 } 69	36 } 74	25 } 60	14 } 66	9 } 54	39
Son or daughter	6	9	20	18	38	35	52	45	30
Other relative	17	14	18	23	17	23	23	28	21
Friend or neighbour	8	4	3	6	7	10	10	7	7
Official of institution	—	—	2	2	2	7	1	11	3
Proportion of respondents in same household as person who died	89%	85%	73%	69%	68%	63%	62%	50%	68%
Number of deaths (=100%)[a]	35	55	145	128	110	112	101	98	785

Age was inadequately recorded on one death certificate.

TABLE A28 *Respondent and the household composition of the person who died*

	On own	*With spouse with or without relatives of the same or an older generation*	*With spouse and relatives of a younger generation*	*With relatives of the same or an older generation*	*With relatives of a younger generation*	*With unrelated people or in guesthouse*
	%	%	%	%	%	%
Husband or wife	—	75	80	—	—	—
Son or daughter	40	12	15	5	77	8
Other relative	38	10	5	85	22	16
Friend or neighbour	22	3	—	10	1	72
Official of institution	—	—	—	—	—	4
Proportion of respondents in same household as person who died	—	76%	93%	60%	87%	60%
Number of deaths (=100%)[a]	100	238	153	40	157	25

[a] Excluding those in hospital or institution for a year or more before their death.

TABLE A29 *Respondent and place of death*

	Place of death (from interview)				
	Hospital	*Other institution*	*Own home*	*Other person's home*	*Elsewhere*
	%	%	%	%	%
Husband or wife	38	10	44	9	46
Son or daughter	29	20	34	30	17
Other relative	22	26	15	61	30
Friend or neighbour	7	8	7	—	7
Official of institution	4	36	—	—	—
Number of deaths (=100%)	365	39	328	23	3

Officials of the institutions were our respondents for just over a third of the people dying there.

We expected that the more closely our respondent was related to the person who died, the more likely they were to be aware of his symptoms and needs, and the more sensitive to his distress. Data in Table A30 generally confirm this, although the differences were not great.

TABLE A30 *Variation in reported needs and symptoms with respondent*

	Husband or wife	*Son or daughter*	*Other relative*	*Unrelated person*	*All respondents*
	%	%	%	%	%
Proportion with a symptom they found very distressing[a]	71	72	67	49	68
Proportion needing help at home with:[b]					
Self care	66	79	63	63	70
Nursing care	57	64	56	44	59
Night care	48	51	40	38	47
Financial help	19	29	20	10	22
Proportion with:	%	%	%	%	%
Pain	72	70	56	53	66
Sleeplessness	54	52	41	38	49
Loss of bladder control	24	38	38	31	32
Loss of bowel control	22	34	28	28	28
Unpleasant smell	11	17	19	19	15
Vomiting	32	32	28	19	30
Loss of appetite	53	46	48	30	48
Constipation	29	35	21	19	28
Bedsores	17	21	14	5	16
Mental confusion	27	45	41	32	36
Trouble with breathing	47	49	41	32	45
Depression	35	39	34	32	36
Other	25	28	23	19	25
No symptoms[a]	14	4	13	8	11
Average number of symptoms	4·3	4·8	4·1	3·3	4·3
Number of deaths (=100%)	303	237	164	81	785

[a] People who died unexpectedly before they were 65 with no previous restrictions have been included as having no symptoms.

[b] Those who had been in hospital or institution for a year or more before they died have been excluded when calculating these percentages.

Close relatives reported more need for personal and night care than people who were less closely related. Friends, neighbours and officials seemed less aware of their needs. The same trend persisted for symptoms such as pain, sleeplessness, loss of appetite and trouble with breathing, but the first three of these were more often reported for people who died at younger ages; so the two factors—age at death and closeness of respondent—might be confounded. Table A31 shows that the closeness of the relationship had an effect within each age group, but the age trends were less clear-cut for particular types of respondent.

TABLE A31 *Variations in reported symptoms with dead person's age and relationship to respondent*

	Husband, wife, son or daughter	*Other respondent*
	Proportion reporting pain	
15–64	73%	59%
65–74	76%	55%
75+	65%	53%
	Proportion reporting sleeplessness	
15–64	55%	43%
65–74	57%	34%
75+	47%	41%
	Proportion reporting loss of appetite	
15–64	55%	53%
65–74	50%	34%
75+	46%	42%
	Proportion reporting trouble breathing	
15–64	43%	45%
65–74	58%	43%
75+	45%	33%
	Number on which percentages based (=100%)	
15–64	180	53
65–74	169	67
75+	187	121

But a number of other symptoms—incontinence, an unpleasant smell and mental confusion—were reported rather less often by husbands and wives than by other respondents, and this was still so within the age groups. Possibly those who were closest to the dying person wanted to deny or forget these unpleasant symptoms, which were likely to be particularly distressing to them personally.

Another apparent effect of not always being able to interview people closely related to the person who died is that we were less likely to get definite answers to some of our questions. For example, when asked if the person who died knew he was unlikely to recover, 17% of the close relatives (husbands, wives and children) were unable to say, whereas 26% of other respondents could give no definite answer. But among those who felt they could say, similar proportions of close relatives and other respondents thought the person knew he was dying.

So in several ways the information we obtained about a person's life in the twelve months before he died was influenced by the closeness of his relationship to the person we were able to interview. It is difficult to see how this problem could be overcome in a comprehensive survey of all deaths, although retrospectively it appears that we might have contacted someone rather more suitable in about 4% of the deaths. In general, the closer the relationship the informant had to the deceased the more sensitive and aware he seemed of the deceased's needs and problems, but there was some evidence that husbands and wives denied the existence of some unpleasant symptoms which they might have felt carried a social stigma; alternatively some of them may have been so used to some symptoms that they did not notice them any more and so failed to report them.

APPENDIX VI

INADEQUATE INFORMATION

Inadequate information may be obtained because the informant does not know or is not prepared to give the information, or because the interviewer does not ask the question, does not probe adequately, or does not record fully. It is often not worthwhile to attempt to distinguish these sources of inadequacy because it is difficult and time-consuming to do so; the numbers are small and the different types of inadequacies are usually treated in the same way—by omitting those for whom inadequate information was obtained and assuming that they were distributed in the same way as the others about whom information is available. Sometimes the fact that the person does not know the answer to a question is a useful piece of information and in that case would be treated separately.

In this survey there were comparatively high numbers of inadequately 'answered' questions. This raises problems of both interpretation and presentation of the results. To know how best to deal with the inadequacies we need to understand the reasons for them and their nature.

Frequency of inadequate information

The proportion of inadequate information at different questions is shown in Table A32.

TABLE A32 *Frequency of inadequate information*

Proportion of inadequate 'responses'	%
None	7
Less than 3%	27
3% but less than 5%	21
5% but less than 10%	26
10% but less than 20%	15
20% or more	4
Number of questions (=100%)	248

Just over half the questions, 55%, were fully completed for 95% or more of the interviews, but one in five of the questions were inadequately answered in 10% or more cases. These proportions are rather rough indications of the size of the problem. On a number of questions which it was expected that some informants would be unable to answer or would be uncertain in their assessments this was allowed for at the pre-codes and codes allocated for this. These have not been included as inadequacies.

The frequency of the inadequacies is higher than that found in other studies made by the Institute. For example, estimates for the proportion of questions with less than 3% inadequacies were about three-fifths on *Parents and Family Planning Services*[1] and four-fifths on *Medicine Takers, Prescribers and Hoarders*[2] compared with about a third on the present study.

Nature of inadequacies

It might be expected that inadequacies more often occurred on questions that were likely to be particularly sensitive—either because the interviewer omitted the question because she felt it might distress the respondent or because she did not 'probe' and ask further questions to clarify unclear responses for the same reason.

Some questions that might be thought potentially distressing to the informant and the proportion for which inadequate information was obtained are given in Table A33.

In fact it did not appear that these questions were particularly inadequately answered.

Inspection of the questions with a high proportion of inadequate 'answers' shows that many of them were 'dependent' questions

TABLE A33 *Potentially distressing questions*

	Proportion of inadequate 'answers'
Did —— know he was not likely to recover? or Did —— know this was likely to happen?	5%
Were you with —— when he died?	1%
How did you feel about —— dying in hospital or institution rather than at home?	3%

[1] Cartwright, Anne, *Parents and Family Planning Services,* unpublished data.

[2] Dunnell, Karen and Cartwright, Anne, *Medicine Takers, Prescribers and Hoarders,* unpublished data.

which only certain groups of informants were asked—depending on their replies to previous questions. All the questions for which 20% or more of the answers were inadequate fell into this category, as did over half of those for which 10%–19% were inadequate. In general it seemed that the more unusual the circumstances, and the less likely the interviewer was to have encountered such a situation before, the more likely she was to obtain inadequate information. For instance, high inadequacy rates, of 15% or more, were obtained for such questions as:

> 'How long had you known him [deceased]?'—which should only have been asked for the 81 respondents who were not relatives.

> 'Did anyone advise him to give up work?'—which should only have been asked about thirty people who died who had retired before they were 65.

Sometimes instructions about when to omit questions seemed over-complicated and were not understood by interviewers. For example, the three questions intended to be omitted only 'if the deceased died at home *and* the informant lived in the same household *or* had not seen the deceased in the last three months' all produced more than 20% inadequate responses.

But just under half of all the questions were dependent ones; so although it looks as if the failure of the interviewers to ask these questions in appropriate circumstances contributed to the high proportion of inadequacies, it is not the only explanation.

The length of the interview and the repetitiveness of some of the questions when the person had needed help with many things also led to omissions.

When we were unable to interview people closely associated with the person who died during the last year of his life, this also contributed to the inadequate replies. For example, the proportion for whom inadequate information was obtained about when they last saw a general practitioner was 4% when a close relative (spouse or child) was interviewed, 11% when it was another relative, and 28% when it was an unrelated person.

On the other hand, inadequate information was more often obtained from relatives than from other informants about whether the person had needed help or more help with different kinds of problems: 18% compared with 11%. Possibly interviewers were reluctant to ask if the respondent thought the person had enough help when the respondent had been involved in caring for the person.

The most serious inadequacy in the data is probably this failure to find out whether people had enough of the various types of help they needed. This was not obtained for 18% of the 6,079 needs for help reported, and when this was summarised for individuals it meant the data were inadequate for 36% of the 656 people needing help.

Handling the problem

This last inadequacy meant that we have been unable to make estimates of the proportion of people reported to need more help than they were given. In other instances we have followed the usual procedure of omitting the inadequate responses and basing estimates just on the people for whom information was obtained. This has meant using a slightly elaborate procedure when the inadequacy related to a dependent question. For example, 37% of the people who died were said to know either probably or certainly that they were going to die—but for 10% of these inadequate information was obtained about who, if anyone, told them this. So to estimate the proportion of all those who died who were told by different people or no one at all we have had to readjust the base to take this into account. In turn this presents a problem of what number to give as the base number. In this situation we have given the larger of the two numbers—that is, including the people for whom inadequate information was available for the dependent question. On other occasions when in theory more than one series of percentages is based on the same number, while in practice different numbers of inadequate answers have had to be excluded, we have given the total number in the group but added a footnote explaining that those for whom inadequate information was available have been excluded when calculating the percentages or averages.

APPENDIX VII

INTERVAL BETWEEN DEATH AND INTERVIEW

Half the sample was chosen from deaths that were registered three months before the interview and the other half from deaths registered nine months before we attempted to contact the relatives. There was no difference in the response rates in the two halves of the sample, but the reasons for the failures were rather different. This is shown in Table A34.

TABLE A34 *Interval and reasons for failures*

	Interval between registration of death and interview	
	Three months	*Nine months*
Refusal	57	40
No one living in the area who could help	19	34
Other	16	9
Total failures	92	83

There were more refusals three months after the death than nine months after, but after the longer interval the reason for the failure was more likely to be that there was no one living in the area, since they had died or moved away.

There was no difference in the type of respondent interviewed: we were as likely to obtain interviews from close relatives nine months after the death as we were three months after the death. But rather more of the respondents interviewed three months after the death said they had helped with arrangements *after* the person died, 54% compared with 45% of those interviewed nine months after. There was no difference in the proportions who had helped *before* death.

Naturally, more of those seen at the nine months' interval had consulted a doctor or nurse since their bereavement, 59% against

42%. In addition, more of the former said they had had a consultation related to their bereavement, 35% compared with 28%. So some people apparently seek professional support for the first time more than three months after they have been bereaved.

One way in which we expected that the information gathered at certain intervals after an event might differ was in the proportion of inadequate or 'uncertain' answers recorded. But this did not seem to have happened generally, although in one instance at any rate the three-month interval seemed to produce more definite answers and stronger feelings. More of those interviewed three months after the person died than of those interviewed nine months after felt it would have been better if the person had died elsewhere—at home if he died in hospital, in hospital if he died at home—and fewer of them were uncertain (see Table A35).

TABLE A35 *Interval and where respondent preferred the deceased to die*

	Interval	
	Three months	*Nine months*
	%	%
Preferred the person to die where he did	70	68
Preferred the person to have died elsewhere	14	8
Respondent uncertain about where preferred person to die	16	24
Number of respondents (=100%)	312	314

A comparison of the interview data with information on the death certificate showed no differences between the two halves of the sample in the extent to which the two sources were in agreement. So the accuracy of the information about the deceased's age, cause of death and place of death did not seem to be affected. Neither were there any significant differences in the symptoms reported for the deceased, their needs for different types of help or the care they were given. One unexplained difference was in the proportion said to have been living alone—18% among those in the three-month sample, 12% in the nine-month.

In general the number and extent of the differences are small.

APPENDIX VIII

STATISTICAL SIGNIFICANCE

There are a number of factors, particularly the nature of the data and the stage at which precise hypotheses are often formulated, which violate some of the conditions in which statistical tests of significance apply and thus make interpretation difficult. For this reason they are rarely referred to in the text, in an attempt to avoid the appearance of spurious precision which the presentation of such tests might seem to imply. But in the absence of more satisfactory techniques these tests have been used to give some indication of the probability of differences occurring by chance.

Chi-square and chi-square trend tests have been applied constantly when looking at the data from this survey. Correlations, t-tests and tests of differences in proportions have also been used. These tests have influenced decisions about what differences to present and how much verbal 'weight' to attach to them. In general, attention has not been drawn to any difference which statistical tests suggest might have occurred by chance five or more times in 100.

Another difficulty about presenting results from a study like this with over 450 items of basic information is that of selection. Inevitably not all cross-analyses are carried out—only about 1,750—and only a fraction of these are presented, which of course gives rise to difficulty in interpreting significance. Positive results are more often shown than negative ones. Readers may sometimes wonder why certain further analyses are not reported. Often, but not always, the analysis will have been done but the result found to be negative or inconclusive.

Table A36 shows the sampling errors for a number of characteristics. Their calculation is based on observed variations in the twelve study areas. For the proportions living alone, the proportion with incontinence and the proportion of people said to have known what was wrong with them, the sampling error is similar to the estimated random sampling error if the sample had been a straight one over the whole country and not just in twelve areas. But for characteristics such as the proportion of deaths at home and the proportion of deaths due to cancer the sampling error is greater than the random one because of the wide variations between areas.

TABLE A36 *Sampling errors*

	Value in total sample	*Range in twelve study areas*	*Sampling error*	*Estimated random sampling error*[a]	*Range: value in total sample ± two sampling errors*
Proportion of deaths in person's own home	39·7%	28·8%–56·3%	2·5%	1·6%	34·7%–44·7%
Proportion of cancer deaths	26·9%	16·3%–45·0%	2·3%	1·4%	22·3%–31·5%
Proportion of deaths of people aged 75 or more	39·7%	21·3%–52·5%	2·8%	1·6%	34·1%–45·3%
Proportion of people who had been in hospital or institution for a year or more before they died	9·2%	0%–20·9%	1·9%	1·0%	5·4%–13·0%
Proportion visited at home by a district nurse[b]	33·3%	22·7%–50·0%	2·6%	1·8%	28·1%–38·5%
Proportion who died, living alone[b]	14·0%	8·2%–21·2%	1·3%	1·3%	11·4%–16·6%
Proportion of people who had loss of bladder control	31·7%	20·8%–46·4%	1·9%	1·7%	27·9%–35·5%
Proportion of people who had loss of bowel control	27·5%	17·5%–35·7%	1·5%	1·6%	24·5%–30·5%
Proportion of people who had loss of bowel and/or bladder control	35·4%	23·6%–50·0%	2·1%	1·7%	31·2%–39·6%
Proportion of people said to have known what was wrong with them	48·8%	39·3%–61·1%	1·8%	1·9%	45·2%–52·4%

[a] If a random sample of country, that is $\sqrt{\frac{p.q.}{n}}$

[b] Excluding those who had been in a hospital or institution for a year or more before they died.

APPENDIX IX

ADDITIONAL DATA ON PEOPLE DYING IN DIFFERENT TYPES OF INSTITUTIONS

These data suggest that people who have been in mental illness hospitals, geriatric hospitals or permanent institutions for a long time appear to be rarely transferred to more acute hospitals for their terminal illness. If they were they would increase the proportion of those dying in the acute hospitals who had been in any hospital or institution for a long time. But, according to the people we interviewed, 55% of those in hospital or an institution for a year or more had been in the same one all the time; 45% had been moved from one hospital or institution to another.

The symptoms reported at the interview for people dying in different types of hospital are shown in Table A38. Pain was least often reported for those dying in mental illness hospitals. Next to those dying in mental illness hospitals, mental confusion was most often reported for those dying in chronic or geriatric hospitals.

These variations in reported symptoms are related to differences in the cause of death and the age at death. These are shown in Table A39.

The proportion dying of cancer was greatest, nearly half in the 'other hospitals'.[1] It was about a third of those dying in private nursing homes or acute hospitals, less than one in ten of those in mental institutions, and one in twenty-five of those in permanent institutions. Deaths from stroke were most common in the chronic long-stay hospitals, private nursing homes and permanent institutions. Deaths from respiratory disease were comparatively rare in acute and partly acute hospitals.

[1] Included in this small group were three, all from the same area, dying in an institution for terminal care, and two, both from another area, who died in one for cancer.

TABLE A37 *Length of stay and type of institution*

<table>
<tr><th rowspan="2">Length of time person had been in any hospital or institution before death</th><th colspan="11">Type of hospital or institution where died (from death certificate)</th><th rowspan="2" colspan="2">All hospitals and institu-tions</th></tr>
<tr><th>Acute</th><th>Partly acute</th><th colspan="2">Geriatric long-stay or chronic</th><th colspan="2">Mental illness</th><th>Other N.H.S. hospitals</th><th>Private hospitals and nursing homes</th><th colspan="2">Permanent institu-tions</th><th></th></tr>
<tr><td></td><td>%</td><td>%</td><td colspan="2">%</td><td colspan="2">%</td><td>%</td><td>%</td><td colspan="2">%</td><td></td><td colspan="2">%</td></tr>
<tr><td>Less than 24 hours</td><td>16</td><td>13</td><td colspan="2">6</td><td colspan="2">—</td><td>3</td><td>16</td><td colspan="2">—</td><td></td><td colspan="2">11</td></tr>
<tr><td>1 day but less than 3 days</td><td>11</td><td>20</td><td colspan="2">4</td><td colspan="2">4</td><td>12</td><td>3</td><td colspan="2">—</td><td></td><td colspan="2">10</td></tr>
<tr><td>3 days but less than 1 week</td><td>16</td><td>15</td><td colspan="2">6</td><td colspan="2">4</td><td>12</td><td>10</td><td colspan="2">5</td><td></td><td colspan="2">12</td></tr>
<tr><td>1 week but less than 1 month</td><td>31</td><td>31</td><td colspan="2">17</td><td colspan="2">8</td><td>24</td><td>13</td><td colspan="2">—</td><td></td><td colspan="2">24</td></tr>
<tr><td>1 month but less than 3 months</td><td>18</td><td>12</td><td colspan="2">16</td><td colspan="2">8</td><td>31</td><td>19</td><td colspan="2">9</td><td></td><td colspan="2">17</td></tr>
<tr><td>3 months but less than 6 months</td><td>6</td><td>6</td><td colspan="2">12</td><td colspan="2">12</td><td>6</td><td>7</td><td colspan="2">4</td><td></td><td colspan="2">7</td></tr>
<tr><td>6 months but less than 1 year</td><td rowspan="4">2</td><td rowspan="4">3</td><td>4</td><td rowspan="4">39</td><td>4</td><td rowspan="4">64</td><td rowspan="4">12</td><td rowspan="4">32</td><td>—</td><td rowspan="4">82</td><td></td><td>1</td><td rowspan="4">19</td></tr>
<tr><td>1 year but less than 2 years</td><td>17</td><td>4</td><td>23</td><td></td><td>5</td></tr>
<tr><td>2 years but less than 5 years</td><td>12</td><td>20</td><td>23</td><td></td><td>7</td></tr>
<tr><td>5 years or more</td><td>6</td><td>36</td><td>36</td><td></td><td>6</td></tr>
<tr><td>Number of deaths (=100%)</td><td>170</td><td>68</td><td colspan="2">51</td><td colspan="2">25</td><td>33</td><td>31</td><td colspan="2">22</td><td></td><td colspan="2">400</td></tr>
</table>

Appendix IX

TABLE A38 *Type of hospital and different types of symptoms*

	Type of hospital or institution				
Symptoms reported at interview	*Acute*	*Partly acute*	*Mental illness*	*Geriatric, long-stay, chronic*	*Other N.H.S. hospitals*
	%	%	%	%	%
Pain	72	77	48	65	79
Sleeplessness	46	44	48	43	58
Loss of bladder control	26	30	44	51	45
Loss of bowel control	22	25	40	43	42
Smell	12	12	24	24	18
Vomiting	30	30	8	20	27
Loss of appetite	49	42	16	35	45
Constipation	28	19	24	29	24
Bedsores	10	8	12	27	18
Mental confusion	36	27	64	59	39
Trouble with breathing	37	53	36	33	52
Depression	41	33	44	29	39
Other	23	33	20	41	36
None[a]	10	11	4	4	6
Number of deaths (=100%)	175	73	25	51	33

[a] Includes those under 65 who died unexpectedly with no previous restrictions. The majority, nine-tenths of those with no symptoms who died in acute hospitals, fell into this category, as did three-quarters of those dying in partly acute hospitals and all those in 'other N.H.S. hospitals'.

TABLE A39 *Type of institution and certified cause of death and age at death*

	Type of institution						
	Acute	*Partly acute*	*Mental illness*	*Geriatric, long-stay, chronic*	*Other N.H.S. hospitals*	*Private hospitals or nursing homes*	*Permanent insti-tutions*
Cause of death (from death certificate)	%	%	%	%	%	%	%
Neoplasm	31	23	8	21	49	36	4
Circulatory	44	52	52	51	24	39	71
Ischaemic heart disease	20	19	28	12	9	7	21
Cerebrovascular disease	17	23	20	29	9	29	29
Other	7	10	4	10	6	3	21
Respiratory	9	12	24	20	18	19	17
Digestive	3	5	4	—	—	—	—
Accident	4	1	8	—	—	3	—
Other	9	7	4	8	9	3	8
Age at death	%	%	%	%	%	%	%
15–44	7	1	—	4	12	6	—
45–54	8	8	—	2	—	6	—
55–64	21	22	16	10	24	6	4
65–69	17	20	8	6	28	23	8
70–74	15	16	4	14	15	20	4
75–79	17	14	36	12	9	3	17
80–84	9	12	16	23	3	16	21
85+	6	7	20	29	9	20	46
Number of deaths in hospitals and institutions (=100%)	176	74	25	51	33	31	24

REFERENCES

ABRAMS, RUTH D., 1970, 'The defences of the terminal cancer patient', Aberdeen, Paper presented at the 2nd International Conference on Social Science and Medicine.

ALDERSON, M. R., 1966, 'Referral to hospital among a representative sample of adults who died', *Proceedings of the Royal Society of Medicine*, 59, pp. 719–21.

ANDERSON, J. A. D. and WARREN, ELIZABETH A., 1966, 'Communications with general practitioners', *Medical Officer*, 116, pp. 333–7.

ASHFORD, J. R. and PEARSON, N. G., 1970, 'Who uses the health services and why?', *Journal of the Royal Statistical Society*, Series A, 133, pp. 295–345.

BOTT, ELIZABETH, 1957, *Family and Social Network*, London, Tavistock.

BRANDON, RUTH, 1972, *Seventy Plus*, British Broadcasting Corporation.

BRAUER, PAUL H., 1965, 'Should the patient be told the truth?', in James K. Skipper and Robert C. Leonard (eds), *Social Interaction and Patient Care*, Philadelphia, J. B. Lippincott, pp. 167–78.

BROCKLEHURST, J. C. and SHERGOLD, MARGARET, 1968, 'What happens when geriatric patients leave hospital?', *Lancet*, ii, pp. 1133–5.

BUCKLE, JUDITH R., 1971, *Work and Housing of Impaired Persons in Great Britain*, London, HMSO.

BUTLER, JOHN R. and PEARSON, MARY, 1970, *Who Goes Home?*, Occasional Papers on Social Administration No. 34, London, G. Bell.

CARSTAIRS, VERA, 1966, *Home Nursing in Scotland*, Scottish Home and Health Department.

CARTWRIGHT, ANN, 1964, *Human Relations and Hospital Care*, London, Routledge & Kegan Paul.

CARTWRIGHT, ANN, 1967, *Patients and their Doctors*, London, Routledge & Kegan Paul.

CARTWRIGHT, ANN, 1970, *Parents and Family Planning Services*, London, Routledge & Kegan Paul.

CHAPLIN, N. W. (ed), 1969, *The Hospitals Year Book*, London, Institute of Hospital Administrators.

CLARKE, MAY, 1969, *Trouble with Feet*, Occasional Papers on Social Administration No. 29, London, G. Bell.

Consumers' Association, 1969, *What to do when someone dies*, London.

DAVIES, BLEDDYN P., BARTON, ANDREW J., MCMILLAN, IAN S. and WILLIAMSON, VALERIE K., 1971, *Variations in Services for the Aged*, Occasional Papers on Social Administration No. 40, London, G. Bell.

Department of Health and Social Security, 1969, *Annual Report for 1968*, London, HMSO.

Department of Health and Social Security and Office of Population

Censuses and Surveys, 1970, *Report on Hospital In-Patient Enquiry for the year 1967. Part 1, Tables*. London, HMSO.

DUFF, RAYMOND S. and HOLLINGSHEAD, AUGUST B., 1968, *Sickness and Society*, London, Harper & Row.

DUNNELL, KAREN and CARTWRIGHT, ANN, 1972, *Medicine Takers, Prescribers and Hoarders*, London, Routledge & Kegan Paul.

EXTON-SMITH, A. N., 1961, 'Terminal illness in the aged', *Lancet*, pp. 305–8.

FERGUSON, T. and MACPHAIL, A. N., 1954, *Hospital and Community*, London, Oxford University Press.

General Register Office, *Annual Reports*, London, HMSO.

General Register Office, 1966, *Classification of Occupations, 1966*, London, HMSO.

General Register Office, 1968, *Sample Census 1966. Household Composition Tables*, London, HMSO.

GILBERTSEN, VICTOR A. and WANGENSTEEN, OWEN H., 1961, 'Should the doctor tell the patient that the disease is cancer?', in *The Physician and the Total Care of the Cancer Patient*, New York, American Cancer Society, pp. 80–5.

GILHORNE, K. R. and NEWELL, D. J., 1972, 'Community services for the elderly', in Gordon McLachlan (ed.), *Problems and Progress in Medical Care*, seventh series, London, Oxford University Press.

GLASER, BARNEY G. and STRAUSS, ANSELM L., 1965, *Awareness of Dying*, London, Weidenfeld & Nicolson.

GLASER, BARNEY G. and STRAUSS, ANSELM L., 1968, *Time for Dying*, Chicago, Aldine.

GOFFMAN, ERVING, 1968, *Asylums*, Harmondsworth, Penguin Books.

GOLDBERG, E. M., *et al.*, 1970, *Helping the Aged*, London, Allen & Unwin.

GOLODETZ, ARNOLD; EVANS, ROSEMARY; HEINRITZ, GRETCHEN and GIBSON JNR, COUNT, D., 1969, 'The care of chronic illness: the "responsor" role', *Medical Care*, 7, pp. 385–94.

GORER, G., 1965, *Death, Grief and Mourning in Contemporary Britain*, London, The Cresset Press.

GREGORY, PETER and YOUNG, MICHAEL, 1972, *Lifeline Telephone Service for the Elderly*, National Innovations Centre.

HARRIS, AMELIA, I., 1968, *Social Welfare for the Elderly, Vol. 1, Comparison of Areas and Summary*, London, HMSO.

HART, JULIAN TUDOR, 1971, 'The inverse care law', *Lancet*, i, pp. 405–12.

HINTON, JOHN, 1967, *Dying*, Harmondsworth, Penguin Books.

HINTON, JOHN, 1970, 'Communication between husband and wife in terminal cancer', Aberdeen, Paper presented at 2nd International Conference on Social Science and Medicine.

HOBSON, WILLIAM and PEMBERTON, JOHN, 1955, *The Health of the Elderly at Home*, London, Butterworth.

HOCKEY, LISBETH, 1966, *Feeling the Pulse*, London, Queen's Institute of District Nursing.

HOCKEY, LISBETH, 1968, *Care in the Balance*, London, Queen's Institute of District Nursing.

HOCKEY, LISBETH, 1970, 'District nurse attached to hospital', in Lisbeth Hockey and Anne Buttimore, *Co-operation in Patient Care*, Queen's Institute of District Nursing, pp. 1–30.

HUGHES, H. L. GLYN, 1960, *Peace at the Last*, London, Calouste Gulbenkian Foundation.

HUNT, AUDREY, 1970, *The Home Help Service in England and Wales*, London, HMSO.

ISAACS, BERNARD, 1971, 'Geriatric patients: do their families care?', *British Medical Journal*, 4, pp. 282–6.

ISAACS, BERNARD; GUNN, JEAN; MCKECHAN, ANDREW; MCMILLAN, ISOBEL and NEVILLE, YVONNE, 1971, 'The Concept of Pre-Death', *Lancet*, i, p. 1115.

ISAACS, BERNARD, LIVINGSTONE, MAUREEN and NEVILLE, YVONNE, 1972, *Survival of the Unfittest*, London, Routledge & Kegan Paul.

JONES, KINGSLEY, 1965, 'Suicide and the hospital service', *British Journal of Psychiatry*, 111, p. 625.

KELLY, W. D. and FRIESSEN, S. R., 1950, 'Do cancer patients want to be told?', *Surgery*, 27, pp. 822–6.

KUBLER-ROSS, ELISABETH, 1970, *On Death and Dying*, London, Tavistock.

LANCE, HILARY, 1971, 'Transport services in general practice. An experiment in five general practices', *Journal of Royal College of General Practitioners*, 21, Supplement No. 3.

LINDEMANN, ERICH, 1944, 'Symptomatology and management of acute grief', *American Journal of Psychiatry*, 101, pp. 141–8.

LOWE, C. R. and MCKEOWN, THOMAS, 1949, 'The care of the chronic sick: I, medical and nursing requirements', *British Journal of Social Medicine*, 3, p. 110.

MARRIS, PETER, 1958, *Widows and their Families*, London, Routledge & Kegan Paul.

MEYRICK, R. L., 1962, 'A geriatric survey in general practice', *Lancet*, ii, pp. 393–5.

MEYRICK, R. L. and COX, A., 1969, 'A geriatric survey repeated', *Lancet*, i, pp. 1146–9.

MOSELEY, L. G., 1968, 'Variations in socio-medical services for the aged', *Social and Economic Administration*, 2, pp. 169–83.

PARKES, C. MURRAY, 1964, 'Effects of bereavement on physical and mental health – a study of the medical records of widows', *British Medical Journal*, 2, pp. 274–9.

PARKES, C. MURRAY, 1964, 'Grief as an illness', *New Society*, 3, No. 80, p. 11.

PARKES, C. MURRAY and BROWN, R. J., 'Health after bereavement', *Psychosomatic Medicine. In Press.*

PARSONS, TALCOTT and BATES, ROBERT F., 1955, *Family Socialization and Interaction Process*, Chicago, Free Press.

PEARSON, LEONARD (ed.), 1969, *Death and Dying*, Cleveland, Case Western Reserve University Press.

REES, W. DEWI and LUTKINS, SYLVIA G., 1967, 'Mortality of bereavement', *British Medical Journal*, 4, pp. 13–16.

The Registrar General, 1971, *Decennial Supplement, England and Wales 1961, Occupational Mortality Tables.*

REIN, MARTIN, 1969, 'Social class and the health service', *New Society*, 14, pp. 807–10.

REIN, MARTIN, 1969, 'Social class and the utilization of medical care services', *Journal of the American Hospitals Association*, 43, pp. 43–54.

SAINSBURY, PETER, 1955, *Suicide in London*, London, Chapman & Hall.

SAUNDERS, CICELY M. S., 1963, 'The treatment of intractable pain in terminal cancer', *Proceedings of the Royal Society of Medicine*, 56, pp. 191–7.

SAUNDERS, CICELY M. S., 1967, 'The care of the terminal stages of cancer', *Annals of the Royal College of Surgeons of England*, 41, Supplement, pp. 162–9.

SAUNDERS, CICELY, M. S., 1969, 'The moment of truth: care of the dying person', in Leonard Pearson (ed.), *Death and Dying*, Cleveland, Case Western Reserve University Press, pp. 49–78.

SEAGER, C. P. and FLOOD, R. A., 1965, 'Suicide in Bristol', *British Journal of Psychiatry*, 111, p. 919.

SHELDON, J. H., 1948, *The Social Medicine of Old Age*, London, Oxford University Press.

TITMUSS, RICHARD M., 1963, *Essays on 'The Welfare State'*, London, Allen & Unwin.

TITMUSS, RICHARD M., 1968, *Commitment to Welfare*, London, Allen & Unwin.

TOWNSEND, PETER, 1957, *The Family Life of Old People*, London, Routledge & Kegan Paul.

TOWNSEND, PETER, 1962, *The Last Refuge*, London, Routledge & Kegan Paul.

TOWNSEND, PETER and WEDDERBURN, DOROTHY, 1965, *The Aged in the Welfare State*, Occasional Papers on Social Administration, No. 14, London, G. Bell.

TUNSTALL, JEREMY, 1966, *Old and Alone*, London, Routledge & Kegan Paul.

VOLKART, EDMUND H. and MICHAEL, STANLEY, T., 1965, 'Bereavement and mental health', in Robert Fulton (ed.), *Death and Identity*, New York, John Wiley, pp. 272–93.

WARREN, M. D., COOPER, J. and WARREN, J. L., 1967, 'Problems of emergency admissions to London hospitals', *British Journal of Preventive and Social Medicine*, 21, pp. 141–9.

WILKES, ERIC, 1965, 'Terminal cancer at home', *Lancet*, i, pp. 799–801.

WILLAMSON, J.; STOKOE, I. H.; GRAY, SALLIE; FISHER, MARY; SMITH, ALWYN; MCGHEE, ANNE and STEPHENSON, ELSIE, 1964, 'Old people at home: their unreported needs', *Lancet*, i, pp. 1117–20.

WILLMOTT, PETER and YOUNG, MICHAEL, 1960, *Family and Class in a London Suburb*, London, Routledge & Kegan Paul.

World Health Organization, 1967, *Manual of the International Statistical Classification of Diseases, Injuries and Causes of Death*, Geneva, WHO.

YOUNG, M.; BENJAMIN, B. and WALLIS, C., 1963, 'The mortality of widowers', *Lancet*, ii, p. 454–6.

INDEX

International Library of Sociology

Edited by

John Rex

University of Warwick

Founded by

Karl Mannheim

as The International Library of Sociology and Social Reconstruction

This Catalogue also contains other Social Science series published by Routledge

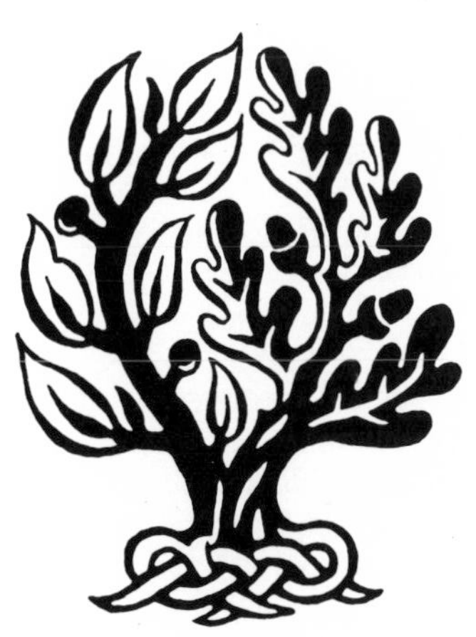

Routledge & Kegan Paul London and Boston

68-74 Carter Lane London EC4V 5EL
9 Park Street Boston Mass 02108

Contents

● *Books so marked are available in paperback*

All books are in Metric Demy 8vo format (216 × 138mm approx.)

GENERAL SOCIOLOGY

Belshaw, Cyril. The Conditions of Social Performance. *An Exploratory Theory. 144 pp.*

Brown, Robert. Explanation in Social Science. *208 pp.*

● Rules and Laws in Sociology.

Cain, Maureen E. Society and the Policeman's Role. *About 300 pp.*

Gibson, Quentin. The Logic of Social Enquiry. *240 pp.*

Gurvitch, Georges. Sociology of Law. *Preface by Roscoe Pound. 264 pp.*

Homans, George C. Sentiments and Activities: *Essays in Social Science. 336 pp.*

Johnson, Harry M. Sociology: *a Systematic Introduction. Foreword by Robert K. Merton. 710 pp.*

Mannheim, Karl. Essays on Sociology and Social Psychology. *Edited by Paul Keckskemeti. With Editorial Note by Adolph Lowe. 344 pp.*

Systematic Sociology: *An Introduction to the Study of Society. Edited by J. S. Erös and Professor W. A. C. Stewart. 220 pp.*

Martindale, Don. The Nature and Types of Sociological Theory. *292 pp.*

● **Maus, Heinz.** A Short History of Sociology. *234 pp.*

Mey, Harald. Field-Theory. *A Study of its Application in the Social Sciences. 352 pp.*

Myrdal, Gunnar. Value in Social Theory: *A Collection of Essays on Methodology. Edited by Paul Streeten. 332 pp.*

Ogburn, William F., and **Nimkoff, Meyer F.** A Handbook of Sociology. *Preface by Karl Mannheim. 656 pp. 46 figures. 35 tables.*

Parsons, Talcott, and **Smelser, Neil J.** Economy and Society: *A Study in the Integration of Economic and Social Theory. 362 pp.*

● **Rex, John.** Key Problems of Sociological Theory. *220 pp.*

Urry, John. Reference Groups and the Theory of Revolution.

FOREIGN CLASSICS OF SOCIOLOGY

● **Durkheim, Emile.** Suicide. *A Study in Sociology. Edited and with an Introduction by George Simpson. 404 pp.*

Professional Ethics and Civic Morals. *Translated by Cornelia Brookfield. 288 pp.*

● **Gerth, H. H.,** and **Mills, C. Wright.** From Max Weber: *Essays in Sociology. 502 pp.*

Tönnies, Ferdinand. Community and Association. *(Gemeinschaft und Gesellschaft.) Translated and Supplemented by Charles P. Loomis. Foreword by Pitirim A. Sorokin. 334 pp.*

SOCIAL STRUCTURE

Andreski, Stanislav. Military Organization and Society. *Foreword by Professor A. R. Radcliffe-Brown. 226 pp. 1 folder.*

Coontz, Sydney H. Population Theories and the Economic Interpretation. *202 pp.*

Coser, Lewis. The Functions of Social Conflict. *204 pp.*

Dickie-Clark, H. F. Marginal Situation: *A Sociological Study of a Coloured Group. 240 pp. 11 tables.*

Glass, D. V. (Ed.). Social Mobility in Britain. *Contributions by J. Berent, T. Bottomore, R. C. Chambers, J. Floud, D. V. Glass, J. R. Hall, H. T. Himmelweit, R. K. Kelsall, F. M. Martin, C. A. Moser, R. Mukherjee, and W. Ziegel. 420 pp.*

Glaser, Barney, and **Strauss, Anselm L.** Status Passage. *A Formal Theory. 208 pp.*

Jones, Garth N. Planned Organizational Change: *An Exploratory Study Using an Empirical Approach. 268 pp.*

Kelsall, R. K. Higher Civil Servants in Britain: *From 1870 to the Present Day. 268 pp. 31 tables.*

König, René. The Community. *232 pp. Illustrated.*

● **Lawton, Denis.** Social Class, Language and Education. *192 pp.*

McLeish, John. The Theory of Social Change: *Four Views Considered. 128 pp.*

Marsh, David C. The Changing Social Structure of England and Wales, 1871-1961. *288 pp.*

Mouzelis, Nicos. Organization and Bureaucracy. *An Analysis of Modern Theories. 240 pp.*

Mulkay, M. J. Functionalism, Exchange and Theoretical Strategy. *272 pp.*

Ossowski, Stanislaw. Class Structure in the Social Consciousness. *210 pp.*

SOCIOLOGY AND POLITICS

Hertz, Frederick. Nationality in History and Politics: *A Psychology and Sociology of National Sentiment and Nationalism. 432 pp.*

Kornhauser, William. The Politics of Mass Society. *272 pp. 20 tables.*

Laidler, Harry W. History of Socialism. *Social-Economic Movements: An Historical and Comparative Survey of Socialism, Communism, Co-operation, Utopianism; and other Systems of Reform and Reconstruction. 992 pp.*

Mannheim, Karl. Freedom, Power and Democratic Planning. *Edited by Hans Gerth and Ernest K. Bramstedt. 424 pp.*

Mansur, Fatma. Process of Independence. *Foreword by A. H. Hanson. 208 pp.*

Martin, David A. Pacificism: *an Historical and Sociological Study. 262 pp.*

Myrdal, Gunnar. The Political Element in the Development of Economic Theory. *Translated from the German by Paul Streeten. 282 pp.*

Wootton, Graham. Workers, Unions and the State. *188 pp.*

FOREIGN AFFAIRS: THEIR SOCIAL, POLITICAL AND ECONOMIC FOUNDATIONS

Mayer, J. P. Political Thought in France from the Revolution to the Fifth Republic. *164 pp.*

CRIMINOLOGY

Ancel, Marc. Social Defence: *A Modern Approach to Criminal Problems. Foreword by Leon Radzinowicz. 240 pp.*

Cloward, Richard A., and **Ohlin, Lloyd E.** Delinquency and Opportunity: *A Theory of Delinquent Gangs. 248 pp.*

Downes, David M. The Delinquent Solution. *A Study in Subcultural Theory. 296 pp.*

Dunlop, A. B., and **McCabe, S.** Young Men in Detention Centres. *192 pp.*

Friedlander, Kate. The Psycho-Analytical Approach to Juvenile Delinquency: *Theory, Case Studies, Treatment. 320 pp.*

Glueck, Sheldon, and **Eleanor.** Family Environment and Delinquency. *With the statistical assistance of Rose W. Kneznek. 340 pp.*

Lopez-Rey, Manuel. Crime. *An Analytical Appraisal. 288 pp.*

Mannheim, Hermann. Comparative Criminology: *a Text Book. Two volumes. 442 pp. and 380 pp.*

Morris, Terence. The Criminal Area: *A Study in Social Ecology. Foreword by Hermann Mannheim. 232 pp. 25 tables. 4 maps.*

● **Taylor, Ian, Walton, Paul,** and **Young, Jock.** The New Criminology. *For a Social Theory of Deviance.*

SOCIAL PSYCHOLOGY

Bagley, Christopher. The Social Psychology of the Epileptic Child. *320 pp.*

Barbu, Zevedei. Problems of Historical Psychology. *248 pp.*

Blackburn, Julian. Psychology and the Social Pattern. *184 pp.*

● **Brittan, Arthur.** Meanings and Situations. *224 pp.*

● **Fleming, C. M.** Adolescence: Its Social Psychology. *With an Introduction to recent findings from the fields of Anthropology, Physiology, Medicine, Psychometrics and Sociometry. 288 pp.*

● The Social Psychology of Education: *An Introduction and Guide to Its Study. 136 pp.*

Homans, George C. The Human Group. *Foreword by Bernard DeVoto. Introduction by Robert K. Merton. 526 pp.*

Social Behaviour: *its Elementary Forms. 416 pp.*

Klein, Josephine. The Study of Groups. *226 pp. 31 figures. 5 tables.*

Linton, Ralph. The Cultural Background of Personality. *132 pp.*

Mayo, Elton. The Social Problems of an Industrial Civilization. *With an appendix on the Political Problem. 180 pp.*

Ottaway, A. K. C. Learning Through Group Experience. *176 pp.*

Ridder, J. C. de. The Personality of the Urban African in South Africa. *A Thematic Apperception Test Study. 196 pp. 12 plates.*

● **Rose, Arnold M.** (Ed.). Human Behaviour and Social Processes: *an Interactionist Approach. Contributions by Arnold M. Rose, Ralph H. Turner, Anselm Strauss, Everett C. Hughes, E. Franklin Frazier, Howard S. Becker, et al. 696 pp.*

Smelser, Neil J. Theory of Collective Behaviour. *448 pp.*
Stephenson, Geoffrey M. The Development of Conscience. *128 pp.*
Young, Kimball. Handbook of Social Psychology. *658 pp. 16 figures. 10 tables.*

SOCIOLOGY OF THE FAMILY

Banks, J. A. Prosperity and Parenthood: *A Study of Family Planning among The Victorian Middle Classes. 262 pp.*
Bell, Colin R. Middle Class Families: *Social and Geographical Mobility. 224 pp.*
Burton, Lindy. Vulnerable Children. *272 pp.*
Gavron, Hannah. The Captive Wife: *Conflicts of Household Mothers. 190 pp.*
George, Victor, and **Wilding, Paul.** Motherless Families. *220 pp.*
Klein, Josephine. Samples from English Cultures.
1. Three Preliminary Studies and Aspects of Adult Life in England. *447 pp.*
2. Child-Rearing Practices and Index. *247 pp.*

Klein, Viola. Britain's Married Women Workers. *180 pp.*
The Feminine Character. *History of an Ideology. 244 pp.*
McWhinnie, Alexina M. Adopted Children. *How They Grow Up. 304 pp.*
Myrdal, Alva, and **Klein, Viola.** Women's Two Roles: *Home and Work. 238 pp. 27 tables.*
Parsons, Talcott, and **Bales, Robert F.** Family: Socialization and Interaction Process. *In collaboration with James Olds, Morris Zelditch and Philip E. Slater. 456 pp. 50 figures and tables.*

SOCIAL SERVICES

Bastide, Roger. The Sociology of Mental Disorder. *Translated from the French by Jean McNeil. 260 pp.*
Carlebach, Julius. Caring For Children in Trouble. *266 pp.*
Forder, R. A. (Ed.). Penelope Hall's Social Services of England and Wales. *352 pp.*
George, Victor. Foster Care. *Theory and Practice. 234 pp.*
Social Security: *Beveridge and After. 258 pp.*
● **Goetschius, George W.** Working with Community Groups. *256 pp.*
Goetschius, George W., and **Tash, Joan.** Working with Unattached Youth. *416 pp.*
Hall, M. P., and **Howes, I. V.** The Church in Social Work. *A Study of Moral Welfare Work undertaken by the Church of England. 320 pp.*
Heywood, Jean S. Children in Care: *the Development of the Service for the Deprived Child. 264 pp.*
Hoenig, J., and **Hamilton, Marian W.** The De-Segration of the Mentally Ill. *284 pp.*
Jones, Kathleen. Mental Health and Social Policy, 1845-1959. *264 pp.*

King, Roy D., Raynes, Norma V., and **Tizard, Jack.** Patterns of Residential Care. *356 pp.*
Leigh, John. Young People and Leisure. *256 pp.*
Morris, Mary. Voluntary Work and the Welfare State. *300 pp.*
Morris, Pauline. Put Away: *A Sociological Study of Institutions for the Mentally Retarded. 364 pp.*
Nokes, P. L. The Professional Task in Welfare Practice. *152 pp.*
Timms, Noel. Psychiatric Social Work in Great Britain (1939-1962). *280 pp.*
● Social Casework: *Principles and Practice. 256 pp.*
Young, A. F., and **Ashton, E. T.** British Social Work in the Nineteenth Century. *288 pp.*
Young, A. F. Social Services in British Industry. *272 pp.*

SOCIOLOGY OF EDUCATION

Banks, Olive. Parity and Prestige in English Secondary Education: a Study in Educational Sociology. *272 pp.*
Bentwich, Joseph. Education in Israel. *224 pp. 8 pp. plates.*
● **Blyth, W. A. L.** English Primary Education. *A Sociological Description.*
1. Schools. *232 pp.*
2. Background. *168 pp.*
Collier, K. G. The Social Purposes of Education: *Personal and Social Values in Education. 268 pp.*
Dale, R. R., and **Griffith, S.** Down Stream: *Failure in the Grammar School. 108 pp.*
Dore, R. P. Education in Tokugawa Japan. *356 pp. 9 pp. plates*
Evans, K. M. Sociometry and Education. *158 pp.*
Foster, P. J. Education and Social Change in Ghana. *336 pp. 3 maps.*
Fraser, W. R. Education and Society in Modern France. *150 pp.*
Grace, Gerald R. Role Conflict and the Teacher. *About 200 pp.*
Hans, Nicholas. New Trends in Education in the Eighteenth Century. *278 pp. 19 tables.*
● Comparative Education: *A Study of Educational Factors and Traditions. 360 pp.*
Hargreaves, David. Interpersonal Relations and Education. *432 pp.*
● Social Relations in a Secondary School. *240 pp.*
Holmes, Brian. Problems in Education. *A Comparative Approach. 336 pp.*
King, Ronald. Values and Involvement in a Grammar School. *164 pp.*
School Organization and Pupil Involvement. *A Study of Secondary Schools.*
● **Mannheim, Karl,** and **Stewart, W. A. C.** An Introduction to the Sociology of Education. *206 pp.*
Morris, Raymond N. The Sixth Form and College Entrance. *231 pp.*
● **Musgrove, F.** Youth and the Social Order. *176 pp.*
● **Ottaway, A. K. C.** Education and Society: An Introduction to the Sociology of Education. *With an Introduction by W. O. Lester Smith. 212 pp.*
Peers, Robert. Adult Education: *A Comparative Study. 398 pp.*

Pritchard, D. G. Education and the Handicapped: *1760 to 1960. 258 pp.*
Richardson, Helen. Adolescent Girls in Approved Schools. *308 pp.*
Stratta, Erica. The Education of Borstal Boys. *A Study of their Educational Experiences prior to, and during Borstal Training. 256 pp.*

SOCIOLOGY OF CULTURE

Eppel, E. M., and **M.** Adolescents and Morality: *A Study of some Moral Values and Dilemmas of Working Adolescents in the Context of a changing Climate of Opinion. Foreword by W. J. H. Sprott. 268 pp. 39 tables.*
● **Fromm, Erich.** The Fear of Freedom. *286 pp.*
The Sane Society. *400 pp.*
Mannheim, Karl. Essays on the Sociology of Culture. *Edited by Ernst Mannheim in co-operation with Paul Kecskemeti. Editorial Note by Adolph Lowe. 280 pp.*
Weber, Alfred. Farewell to European History: *or The Conquest of Nihilism Translated from the German by R. F. C. Hull. 224 pp.*

SOCIOLOGY OF RELIGION

Argyle, Michael. Religious Behaviour. *224 pp. 8 figures. 41 tables.*
Nelson, G. K. Spiritualism and Society. *313 pp.*
Stark, Werner. The Sociology of Religion. *A Study of Christendom.*
Volume I. *Established Religion. 248 pp.*
Volume II. *Sectarian Religion. 368 pp.*
Volume III. *The Universal Church. 464 pp.*
Volume IV. *Types of Religious Man. 352 pp.*
Volume V. *Types of Religious Culture. 464 pp.*
Watt, W. Montgomery. Islam and the Integration of Society. *320 pp.*

SOCIOLOGY OF ART AND LITERATURE

Jarvie, Ian C. Towards a Sociology of the Cinema. *A Comparative Essay on the Structure and Functioning of a Major Entertainment Industry. 405 pp.*
Rust, Frances S. Dance in Society. *An Analysis of the Relationships between the Social Dance and Society in England from the Middle Ages to the Present Day. 256 pp. 8 pp. of plates.*
Schücking, L. L. The Sociology of Literary Taste. *112 pp.*

SOCIOLOGY OF KNOWLEDGE

Mannheim, Karl. Essays on the Sociology of Knowledge. *Edited by Paul Kecskemeti. Editorial Note by Adolph Lowe. 353 pp.*

Remmling, Gunter W. (Ed.). Towards the Sociology of Knowledge. *Origins and Development of a Sociological Thought Style.*

Stark, Werner. The Sociology of Knowledge: *An Essay in Aid of a Deeper Understanding of the History of Ideas. 384 pp.*

URBAN SOCIOLOGY

Ashworth, William. The Genesis of Modern British Town Planning: *A Study in Economic and Social History of the Nineteenth and Twentieth Centuries. 288 pp.*

Cullingworth, J. B. Housing Needs and Planning Policy: *A Restatement of the Problems of Housing Need and 'Overspill' in England and Wales. 232 pp. 44 tables. 8 maps.*

Dickinson, Robert E. City and Region: *A Geographical Interpretation. 608 pp. 125 figures.*

The West European City: *A Geographical Interpretation. 600 pp. 129 maps. 29 plates.*

● The City Region in Western Europe. *320 pp. Maps.*

Humphreys, Alexander J. New Dubliners: *Urbanization and the Irish Family. Foreword by George C. Homans. 304 pp.*

Jackson, Brian. Working Class Community: *Some General Notions raised by a Series of Studies in Northern England. 192 pp.*

Jennings, Hilda. Societies in the Making: *a Study of Development and Redevelopment within a County Borough. Foreword by D. A. Clark. 286 pp.*

● **Mann, P. H.** An Approach to Urban Sociology. *240 pp.*

Morris, R. N., and **Mogey, J.** The Sociology of Housing. *Studies at Berinsfield. 232 pp. 4 pp. plates.*

Rosser, C., and **Harris, C.** The Family and Social Change. *A Study of Family and Kinship in a South Wales Town. 352 pp. 8 maps.*

RURAL SOCIOLOGY

Chambers, R. J. H. Settlement Schemes in Tropical Africa: *A Selective Study. 268 pp.*

Haswell, M. R. The Economics of Development in Village India. *120 pp.*

Littlejohn, James. Westrigg: *the Sociology of a Cheviot Parish. 172 pp. 5 figures.*

Mayer, Adrian C. Peasants in the Pacific. *A Study of Fiji Indian Rural Society. 248 pp. 20 plates.*

Williams, W. M. The Sociology of an English Village: *Gosforth. 272 pp. 12 figures. 13 tables.*

SOCIOLOGY OF INDUSTRY AND DISTRIBUTION

Anderson, Nels. Work and Leisure. *280 pp.*

● **Blau, Peter M.,** and **Scott, W. Richard.** Formal Organizations: *a Comparative approach. Introduction and Additional Bibliography by J. H. Smith. 326 pp.*

Eldridge, J. E. T. Industrial Disputes. *Essays in the Sociology of Industrial Relations. 288 pp.*

Hetzler, Stanley. Applied Measures for Promoting Technological Growth. *352 pp.*

Technological Growth and Social Change. *Achieving Modernization. 269 pp.*

Hollowell, Peter G. The Lorry Driver. *272 pp.*

Jefferys, Margot, *with the assistance of Winifred Moss.* Mobility in the Labour Market: *Employment Changes in Battersea and Dagenham. Preface by Barbara Wootton. 186 pp. 51 tables.*

Millerson, Geoffrey. The Qualifying Associations: *a Study in Professionalization. 320 pp.*

Smelser, Neil J. Social Change in the Industrial Revolution: *An Application of Theory to the Lancashire Cotton Industry, 1770-1840. 468 pp. 12 figures. 14 tables.*

Williams, Gertrude. Recruitment to Skilled Trades. *240 pp.*

Young, A. F. Industrial Injuries Insurance: *an Examination of British Policy. 192 pp.*

DOCUMENTARY

Schlesinger, Rudolf (Ed.). Changing Attitudes in Soviet Russia.

2. The Nationalities Problem and Soviet Administration. *Selected Readings on the Development of Soviet Nationalities Policies. Introduced by the editor. Translated by W. W. Gottlieb. 324 pp.*

ANTHROPOLOGY

Ammar, Hamed. Growing up in an Egyptian Village: *Silwa, Province of Aswan. 336 pp.*

Brandel-Syrier, Mia. Reeftown Elite. *A Study of Social Mobility in a Modern African Community on the Reef. 376 pp.*

Crook, David, and **Isabel.** Revolution in a Chinese Village: *Ten Mile Inn. 230 pp. 8 plates. 1 map.*

Dickie-Clark, H. F. The Marginal Situation. *A Sociological Study of a Coloured Group. 236 pp.*

Dube, S. C. Indian Village. *Foreword by Morris Edward Opler. 276 pp. 4 plates.*

India's Changing Villages: *Human Factors in Community Development. 260 pp. 8 plates. 1 map.*

Firth, Raymond. Malay Fishermen. *Their Peasant Economy. 420 pp. 17 pp. plates.*

Gulliver, P. H. Social Control in an African Society: a Study of the Arusha, Agricultural Masai of Northern Tanganyika. *320 pp. 8 plates. 10 figures.*

Ishwaran, K. Shivapur. *A South Indian Village. 216 pp.*

Tradition and Economy in Village India: *An Interactionist Approach. Foreword by Conrad Arensburg. 176 pp.*

Jarvie, Ian C. The Revolution in Anthropology. *268 pp.*

Jarvie, Ian C., and **Agassi, Joseph.** Hong Kong. *A Society in Transition. 396 pp. Illustrated with plates and maps.*

Little, Kenneth L. Mende of Sierra Leone. *308 pp. and folder.*

Negroes in Britain. *With a New Introduction and Contemporary Study by Leonard Bloom. 320 pp.*

Lowie, Robert H. Social Organization. *494 pp.*

Mayer, Adrian C. Caste and Kinship in Central India: *A Village and its Region. 328 pp. 16 plates. 15 figures. 16 tables.*

Smith, Raymond T. The Negro Family in British Guiana: *Family Structure and Social Status in the Villages. With a Foreword by Meyer Fortes. 314 pp. 8 plates. 1 figure. 4 maps.*

SOCIOLOGY AND PHILOSOPHY

Barnsley, John H. The Social Reality of Ethics. *A Comparative Analysis of Moral Codes. 448 pp.*

Diesing, Paul. Patterns of Discovery in the Social Sciences. *362 pp.*

Douglas, Jack D. (Ed.). Understanding Everyday Life. *Toward the Reconstruction of Sociological Knowledge. Contributions by Alan F. Blum. Aaron W. Cicourel, Norman K. Denzin, Jack D. Douglas, John Heeren, Peter McHugh, Peter K. Manning, Melvin Power, Matthew Speier, Roy Turner, D. Lawrence Wieder, Thomas P. Wilson and Don H. Zimmerman. 370 pp.*

Jarvie, Ian C. Concepts and Society. *216 pp.*

Roche, Maurice. Phenomenology, Language and the Social Sciences. *About 400 pp.*

Sahay, Arun. Sociological Analysis.

Sklair, Leslie. The Sociology of Progress. *320 pp.*

International Library of Anthropology

General Editor Adam Kuper

Brown, Raula. The Chimbu. *A Study of Change in the New Guinea Highlands.*

Van Den Berghe, Pierre L. Power and Privilege at an African University.

International Library of Social Policy

General Editor Kathleen Jones

Holman, Robert. Trading in Children. *A Study of Private Fostering.*
Jones, Kathleen. History of the Mental Health Services. *428 pp.*
Thomas, J. E. The English Prison Officer since 1850: *A Study in Conflict. 258 pp.*

Primary Socialization, Language and Education

General Editor Basil Bernstein

Bernstein, Basil. Class, Codes and Control. *2 volumes.*
1. *Theoretical Studies Towards a Sociology of Language. 254 pp.*
2. *Applied Studies Towards a Sociology of Language. About 400 pp.*

Brandis, Walter, and **Henderson, Dorothy.** Social Class, Language and Communication. *288 pp.*
Cook-Gumperz, Jenny. Social Control and Socialization. *A Study of Class Differences in the Language of Maternal Control.*
Gahagan, D. M., and **G. A.** Talk Reform. *Exploration in Language for Infant School Children. 160 pp.*
Robinson, W. P., and **Rackstraw, Susan, D. A.** A Question of Answers. *2 volumes. 192 pp. and 180 pp.*
Turner, Geoffrey, J., and **Mohan, Bernard, A.** A Linguistic Description and Computer Programme for Children's Speech. *208 pp.*

Reports of the Institute of Community Studies

Cartwright, Ann. Human Relations and Hospital Care. *272 pp.*
Parents and Family Planning Services. *306 pp.*
Patients and their Doctors. *A Study of General Practice. 304 pp.*
● **Jackson, Brian.** Streaming: *an Education System in Miniature. 168 pp.*
Jackson, Brian, and **Marsden, Dennis.** Education and the Working Class: *Some General Themes raised by a Study of 88 Working-class Children in a Northern Industrial City. 268 pp. 2 folders.*
Marris, Peter. The Experience of Higher Education. *232 pp. 27 tables.*
Marris, Peter, and **Rein, Martin.** Dilemmas of Social Reform. *Poverty and Community Action in the United States. 256 pp.*
Marris, Peter, and **Somerset, Anthony.** African Businessmen. *A Study of Entrepreneurship and Development in Kenya. 256 pp.*
Mills, Richard. Young Outsiders: *a Study in Alternative Communities.*

Runciman, W. G. Relative Deprivation and Social Justice. *A Study of Attitudes to Social Inequality in Twentieth Century England. 352 pp.*

Townsend, Peter. The Family Life of Old People: *An Inquiry in East London. Foreword by J. H. Sheldon. 300 pp. 3 figures. 63 tables.*

Willmott, Peter. Adolescent Boys in East London. *230 pp.*

The Evolution of a Community: *a study of Dagenham after forty years. 168 pp. 2 maps.*

Willmott, Peter, and **Young, Michael.** Family and Class in a London Suburb. *202 pp. 47 tables.*

Young, Michael. Innovation and Research in Education. *192 pp.*

● **Young, Michael,** and **McGeeney, Patrick.** Learning Begins at Home. *A Study of a Junior School and its Parents. 128 pp.*

Young, Michael, and **Willmott, Peter.** Family and Kinship in East London. *Foreword by Richard M. Titmuss. 252 pp. 39 tables.*

The Symmetrical Family.

Reports of the Institute for Social Studies in Medical Care

Cartwright, Ann, Hockey, Lisbeth, and **Anderson, John L.** Life Before Death.

Dunnell, Karen, and **Cartwright, Ann.** Medicine Takers, Prescribers and Hoarders. *190 pp.*

Medicine, Illness and Society

General Editor W. M. Williams

Robinson, David. The Process of Becoming Ill.

Stacey, Margaret. *et al.* Hospitals, Children and Their Families. *The Report of a Pilot Study. 202 pp.*

Monographs in Social Theory

General Editor Arthur Brittan

Bauman, Zygmunt. Culture as Praxis.

Dixon, Keith. Sociological Theory. *Pretence and Possibility.*

Smith, Anthony D. The Concept of Social Change. *A Critique of the Functionalist Theory of Social Change.*

Routledge Social Science Journals

The British Journal of Sociology. *Edited by Terence P. Morris. Vol. 1, No. 1, March 1950 and Quarterly. Roy. 8vo. Back numbers available. An international journal with articles on all aspects of sociology.*

Economy and Society. *Vol. 1, No. 1. February 1972 and Quarterly. Metric Roy. 8vo. A journal for all social scientists covering sociology, philosophy, anthropology, economics and history. Back numbers available.*

Year Book of Social Policy in Britain, The. *Edited by Kathleen Jones. 1971. Published Annually.*

Printed in Great Britain by Lewis Reprints Limited
Brown Knight & Truscott Group, London and Tonbridge

1373